FREE FOR ALL

FREE FOR ALL

Why the NHS is Worth Saving

GAVIN FRANCIS

PROFILE BOOKS
wellcome collection

First published in Great Britain in 2023 by
Profile Books Ltd
29 Cloth Fair
London
ECIA 7JQ

www.profilebooks.com

Published in association with Wellcome Collection

**wellcome
collection**

183 Euston Road
London NW1 2BE
www.wellcomecollection.org

1 3 5 7 9 10 8 6 4 2

Typeset in Dante by MacGuru Ltd
Printed and bound in Great Britain by
CPI Group (UK) Ltd, Croydon, CR0 4YY

A CIP catalogue record for this book is available from the British Library.

ISBN 978 1 80081 925 2
eISBN 978 1 80081 926 9

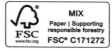

for my colleagues,
whose many unnoticed acts of
kindness and professionalism
sustain the NHS

CONTENTS

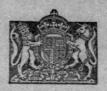

THE NEW
NATIONAL
HEALTH
SERVICE

*

Your new National Health Service begins on 5th July. What is it? How do you get it?

It will provide you with all medical, dental, and nursing care. Everyone—rich or poor, man, woman or child—can use it or any part of it. There are no charges, except for a few special items. There are no insurance qualifications. But it is not a "charity". You are all paying for it, mainly as taxpayers, and it will relieve your money worries in time of illness.

This book has been inspired by hundreds of conversations with dozens of fellow clinicians who work across the NHS. Many of them have preferred to remain anonymous. Names and identifying features of the patient stories that follow have all been changed, but I'd like to reassure the reader that everything described in this book *has happened*, though not to the patient described. Just as physicians must honour the privileged access they have to our bodies, they must honour the trust with which we share our stories. As a doctor who is also a writer, I've spent a great deal of time deliberating over what can and cannot be said without betraying the confidence of my patients. Protecting confidences is an essential part of what I do: 'confidence' means 'with faith' – we are all patients sooner or later; we all want faith that we'll be heard, and that our privacy will be respected.

1

A DAY IN THE LIFE OF (POTENTIALLY) THE BEST JOB IN THE WORLD

An ordinary Tuesday morning and I'm arriving at my GP practice for a day's work. It's 8.30 a.m., and the receptionist on duty is Nicola. 'Any dramas?' I ask her as I approach the desk; 'Not yet, but it's early,' she says with a wry laugh. From the moment the phones begin to ring in the morning until they hand over to the evening service at 6 p.m., practice receptionists are at the front line of the health service, bearing the brunt of patients' anger, disappointment and frustrations with the NHS. A couple of years ago I stopped saying 'good morning' and began to experiment with alternative, more optimistic greetings. 'It's going to be a Tuesday of Happiness,' I say as I stop at the desk. 'Let's hope so!' she replies.

I leave a cup of tea cooling as I switch on the computer, which runs on an old operating system and usually takes a few minutes to get going. The GP computer systems don't talk to the hospital systems, and it often feels for clinicians as if they're drowning in passwords and glitches. Some parts of the NHS still use pagers and, until very recently, fax machines. Most of us are trying to provide medical care fit for the 2020s with computer systems better suited to the 1990s.

There are two letters with handwritten sticky notes laid over my computer keyboard – urgent messages left by colleagues for me to action today. Modern healthcare is so complicated that no one case or story could illustrate the problems of today's NHS, but these two letters, left out for my urgent attention, illustrate some of the pressures on the health service today.

One is a discharge letter about Helen R., a former schoolteacher and a formidable bridge player, a widow and a Londoner, now in her early eighties, who I'd admitted to hospital three weeks earlier for treatment of a kidney infection. The infection had made her confused and unsteady, and she waited most of the day for an ambulance, getting progressively unwell. In the first hours of her admission she'd fallen out of bed onto the hard hospital floor and broken her hip. I know from speaking to hospital colleagues that at the time she fell the ward had been very short of nurses. I feel a flash of guilt, as if I'd broken her hip, though I'd had no choice other than to send her in – the acute medical unit had been the only option open to me to keep her 'safe'. But because of understaffing the hospital ward had proven anything but safe.

The other letter was about William S., a man in his late forties who had been referred for colonoscopy after coming to see one of my colleagues several months ago and complaining of persistent diarrhoea and blood loss, with a discomfort in his lower belly. He had been anxious that his new symptoms were a sign of bowel cancer, and my colleague had referred him urgently for specialist assessment. But because of his relative youth (under fifty-five), and the huge pressures on the service caused in part by pandemic backlog and in part by lack of staff, that referral had been downgraded from 'urgent' to 'routine', and he had waited many months for the test. Now the colonoscopy confirmed what William had most feared: cancer. It had most likely spread to the liver, and a hospital appointment had been scheduled for the following week to discuss what treatment options remained to him. I groaned inwardly and made a note to call William later, to see how he was taking the news. Pressures on the service are now so extreme that urgent referrals are often downgraded, and life-threatening diagnoses are being missed.

The computer seems to be working reasonably well, so I open the four different applications I need to access the different elements of my patients' notes. There are thirty-five pieces of correspondence to read – specialist letters, scans, X-ray reports – and two screen-fuls of blood tests to review. When there's adequate time in the day I enjoy going through these letters, reports and results: they tell me whether the working diagnoses I've made have been correct, and where a test or scan result is unexpected they offer learning points. Special-ist letters help me to plan my next encounters with each patient, and unanticipated results feel like puzzles to be solved, not unwelcome irritations. But on pressured days those anom-alous results feel like obstacles, slowing me down when there's already insufficient time to get through the workload. Hurry creeps in; the chance of things being missed begins to rise. Many of the letters will need to wait until lunchtime to be read properly, but before clinic starts I cherry-pick some easy issues that can be dealt with swiftly.

Only when I've scanned the correspondence do I open my NHS email. A motley collection: one message tells me that the hospice is closed to new admissions, and the community palliative care nurses are struggling to cope. They ask that I avoid referring all but the most complex cases their way, and handle the rest on my own. If any dying patients are in crisis they'll need to be admitted through A&E. There's an email too from the clinical leader of primary care to let me know that the front door of the local hospital is experiencing 'extreme pressure', urging me to explore all possible alternatives before considering an admission for any of my patients – as if I didn't do that already. The tone of the letter is apologetic; this particular clinical leader still works as a GP, and knows how frustrating and patronising these letters seem. The community psychiatry team has rebuffed one of my urgent referrals, and asked me to follow up a suicidal patient myself as they have no capacity to see her. I forward the email to the receptionists, and ask them to find out if the patient can come in today and be added on to the end of my already full clinic.

The local hospital for children has put out a message to say that if any GPs would like to order blood tests for a child, there's a three-month 'wait for an appointment at the local dedicated paediatric clinic – a service so slow that it might as well not exist. I don't make the decision to send children for blood tests lightly, and I can't think of a situation where I'd be happy to wait three months for a result. The children's phlebotomy clinic was set up with good intentions: its staff are highly skilled, and children are less likely to develop a needle phobia if the blood is taken there, rather than by a rushed GP. But it's another example of an underfunded service that has failed to keep up with demand.

There's a letter from Scotland's Chief Medical Officer reminding me that the NHS should not be providing any pre- or post-operative care for people seeking private surgery abroad. The diminution and degradation of the NHS means that health tourism is booming – but so is the cost of fixing foreign hospitals' mistakes. The NHS is still trying to figure out a reliable mechanism to bill overseas private providers for the follow-up required when British people fly abroad for procedures that go wrong.

Only then do I examine the list of the morning's patients. I've been a GP for eighteen years, a partner in this practice for thirteen of those, and about half of the fourteen names are familiar to me. It's the enormous diversity that I love about the work – from the names on the screen, I know I'll be dipping into training in psychiatry, paediatrics, orthopaedics, gynaecology, dermatology, geriatrics, and that the morning will bring problems that, at one end of the spectrum seem fleeting and trivial (though they may not seem so to the patient), and at the other, life-threatening and desperate. Both extremes can be satisfying to treat: in its essence, the practice of medicine is about using medical knowledge to ease suffering, and its best manifestations are a strange alchemy of science and kindness. Even the most seemingly trivial encounter will require me to sift through the patient's story and symptoms for worrying features, excluding scores of potential diagnoses before arriving at the most likely and then formulating a plan that acknowledges the limits of the service and the patient's own preferences.

The architect of the NHS, Aneurin Bevan, wrote of general practice: 'What is not so obvious is that the average doctor is equipped by his general education and by temperament to make an assessment of so many imponderables. He requires for this delicate task imaginative sympathy, sensitivity, and a liberal education.' Doctors and nurse practitioners are obliged to train for a great many years because as a society we expect them to hold a wealth of knowledge about the body and mind, and to exercise wisdom, kindness and professionalism in how they apply it. The enormity of twenty-first century medicine, with its increasingly unwieldy power to diagnose and treat but also to complicate and *over*treat, looms over every encounter. Sometimes it seems absurd to me that so many expectations, or 'imponderables' as Bevan put it, have to be attended to in less than ten minutes. But though my days are always pressured for time, it still feels as if the job is worthwhile, and usually that it's possible to do a great deal of good.

The clinic begins with someone suffering

stomach pains that won't respond to treatment;
her ultrasound scan was normal but her pains
persist; she has been told that it's more than a
year until she'll be seen in the outpatient clinic
and can be considered for an endoscopy. She's
lucky; for some specialties the waiting list to
be seen is now more than two years. Another
patient is just out of hospital after a chaotic
four-day stay; she has two contradictory discharge letters about the plan for treatment
now that she's home, and no hospital follow-up
booked. We spend much of the appointment
time on the phone trying to get through to the
responsible consultant's secretary. One man
has had surgery overseas, and brings a list of
expectations for follow-up, as well as further
tests, all drafted by a doctor whose first language isn't English, and who works in a health
system geared entirely towards profit. I have to
explain that the procedure he paid for wouldn't
have been recommended here in the UK, and
that the follow-up specified by the foreign clinician won't be possible on the NHS – he'll have
to fly back to the country where he got his

surgery if he wants it. He blusters out of the room in anger, and I take a few deep breaths to calm myself before calling the next patient.

One man who speaks no English has missed his long-awaited specialist review because the appointment letter arrived at his home the day after he was due to be seen. I get back on the phone to the secretaries, trying to rearrange the appointment and make sure that the new one will have an interpreter available. Scattered among these complex, difficult conversations are far easier encounters where brief advice, or a simple prescription, have a good chance of curing someone's problem, or at least improving their quality of life: an ear infection, a steroid injection to an arthritic knee, a new cream for scarring acne, HRT for debilitating hot flushes. At the end of the surgery I call William S., and listen for a few minutes to his justified fury at the delayed diagnosis of cancer that now threatens his life. I tell him we'll do everything we can as a practice to support him through the surgery and chemotherapy he now needs.

Among the home visits to be done over lunchtime are an elderly man with paralysing anxiety and chest pains. Since the lockdowns of the pandemic he has been too frightened to leave his house, and his history of heart disease means I'll have to see him at his home to decide whether the pain might be coming from his heart, or whether it's a resurgence of his anxiety. When time is short the temptation to admit to hospital directly for blood tests and an ECG is strong, but I resist it – bad for the patient as well as for the overwhelmed A&E. The other home visit of the day is to Helen R., home now with a replacement of the hip that was broken when she fell on the ward. The joint has been repaired, but she is now unable to walk. The visit is to see whether we can better manage her pain, and assess whether there is enough care coming in from social services to keep her clean and fed. She sits in her front room, heating on low to save money, a blanket over her knees and a woolly hat on her head. 'Mustn't grumble,' she says in her Cockney accent, 'but I don't think I can stick this, sitting here on my own. Do you think I should move into a home?' We spend a while talking about local sheltered housing, and whether one of them might suit her better than a care home.

On my way back to the surgery I buy a sandwich to be eaten at my desk while going through the rest of the correspondence. The local university disability service has written to me about a patient with suspected attention deficit disorder, asking that I write a one-page summary of the difficulties he is having and how the university should adapt their expectations. There are two insurance forms to fill in, and a request for a medical supporting letter for someone's benefits application. Gastroenterology, cardiology, neurology, rheumatology – each of these specialties has its own language, and its own expectations of how I, in the community, might take pressure off their service by doing more for our mutual patient. I go through each of them arranging prescription changes, follow-up appointments and new blood tests based on the letters' recommendations. Clinical colleagues in hospital

understandably want me to do more in the
interests of economy and convenience for the
patient, but it's extremely rare that I receive a
letter asking me to do less, or prescribe less.
It's always more. The cumulative effect of all
these requests, and the frailty of an ageing
population, as well as rising expectations of
what medicine can do, all contribute to making
my days much busier than they were when I
started as a GP two decades ago. Primary care
conducts about 90 per cent of the encounters
in today's NHS, and it does it with less than 10
per cent of the funding. It's a very efficient way
of offering medical care – good for patients and
good for taxpayers, but it's been starved of the
funding required to do what the people, politicians and specialists are now asking of it. Most
GPs passionately want to do the best by their
patients and are crying out for ways of making
their workload more sustainable.

That afternoon I attend a meeting of
doctors from all the GP practices in my sector
of the city. We don't get together very often
because we've all got far too much clinical

work to do. While hospital doctor numbers have been rising steadily, there are 10 per cent fewer GPs now in real terms than there were in 2015, though the number of appointments offered has increased. Many practices in the area are folding – some because they can't recruit replacement staff, others because the antiquated system whereby GPs must provide their own premises doesn't work any more. When GPs get together there's often a great deal of moaning, but there's laughter too – most of us still enjoy helping our patients, and want to find ways of making the system work more sustainably.

None of the GPs in our group have any experience in managing the colossal budgets wielded by the twenty-first-century NHS – we're clinicians, not managers. You would have thought that having spent a minimum of ten years training in clinical medicine (and often as many as twenty years) would mean that we'd self-selected against wanting to manage budgets, but that is exactly what the government believes we should aspire to do. There was a vogue a few years ago for encouraging GPs to sign up for 'leadership training' and 'resilience training', as well as workshops on 'managing change'. That has diminished now as the profession drops into survival mode. I was never sure anyway who was expected to go on seeing the patients while GPs took on these new roles.

The principal speaker was a well-known, widely respected, energetic and accessible consultant physician who has been charged with redesigning elements of how we manage the mounting numbers of frail elderly patients who shuttle back and forth between home and hospital. In my area, the total number of beds available for inpatient care across all specialties has dropped more than 20 per cent since 2003, while the city's population has increased by 25 per cent. The consultant physician told us about plans, already in place, to drop the number of beds available by a further 10 to 15 per cent. 'We can do this,' he said; '40 per cent of the patients in my ward don't need to be there.' This last statistic he quoted with a note of irritation, as if the paucity of beds was somehow our fault as GPs for admitting people in the first place. 'What are you going to do,' he asked us, 'when you phone to admit a patient and we refuse to take them. Because we've no beds. Because there isn't enough money.'

There was a surprised silence. This was new: a senior clinician, involved at the highest level of strategic planning, stating that the system as it stands is on the verge of collapse, and explicitly shifting responsibility for the problem back to general practice, which is itself in deep crisis. Hospital managers are fond of talking about 'bed blockers', and it seems they were now contemplating the relief of blocked beds by refusing admissions. To use a plumbing analogy: if you were to ask a plumber what to do about a blockage, he'd be unlikely to forbid the opening of taps.

Being a GP is potentially the best job in the world: it involves meeting people of every kind, listening to their stories, diagnosing their difficulties, and coming up with plans to improve the quality of their lives. For the entirety of my professional career the state has paid me to do that, and it, in turn, has expected me to act with integrity and professionalism, in the best interests of my patient. But it's getting harder and harder to do that job the way I was trained to do it, and more and more of my days are spent not in helping my patients feel better, but in helping them navigate a failing system.

For a patient to be seen by a GP costs about £38, to be seen in A&E costs about £200, while to call out an ambulance costs around £400. GPs offer more than 300 million consultations per year, while A&E, overwhelmed as it is, has just 23 million patient encounters. If even a fraction of the patients currently seen by GPs end up at the doors of the hospitals, those hospitals will be swamped. The current algorithms used by NHS Direct trigger about double the number of ambulance call-outs as GPs do when taking the same call – computers don't make good doctors. Another reason the ambulance service is overwhelmed has to do with patient perceptions of what constitutes an emergency: one paramedic told me recently that he was called out for a 'bleeding wound' that on arrival proved to be a paper cut.

The National Health Service is an amazing institution, and almost unique in the world. Our country even chose it as the centrepiece of its Olympic opening ceremony in 2012 (though in terms of the quality provided by the service, 2012 now feels like a very long time ago, and it's difficult to imagine an Olympic opening ceremony in 2023 doing the same). That we still have a system the same for everyone, free for all at the point of contact regardless of means, is something worth celebrating and protecting. But the NHS is not working the way it was intended to.

I'm relieved that there's an ongoing national debate about the problems of the NHS, and about how they might be solved for people like you and me, for my patients Helen R. and William S., for the 67 million people of the UK as well as for the approximately 1.4 million people who work within the health service across the four nations. My intention with this book is to make a modest contribution to that debate: to bring it up to the minute with stories that illustrate how poorly it is working right now, offer some suggestions for how things could so easily be better, and passionately defend it as an institution worth saving. It will celebrate the NHS's founding principles because they're good for patients, good for communities and good for my clinical colleagues – good for everyone except private company shareholders.

2

IN PLACE OF FEAR: THE ORIGINS OF THE NHS

With each year that goes by I have fewer patients who remember life before the NHS. One woman remembers her mother keeping a jar of money 'for the doctor' – they never took holidays, and any spare cash was put aside for medical fees. Another told me that her family made do with visits to the herbalist's shop – herbal medicines were less effective than pharmaceuticals but more affordable. Illness could ruin a family's prospects, and frequently did; healthcare for the poor was distributed through churches and charitable foundations with patchy coverage. In 1800, one in three babies born in Britain would die before the age of five; by 1930 that figure was still as high as one in ten. Public health improvements have led to a steady downward trend ever since – one of the steepest drops was between 1945 and 1950 when the introduction of the NHS saw child mortality drop by 32 per cent. In 1950 the UK was in the top six countries for life expectancy worldwide – only the Dutch and the Scandinavians lived longer. By 2015 the UK had slipped to twenty-first in terms of life expectancy, and by 2021 it had fallen to thirty-seventh, not solely because of the pandemic but because of political decisions about the funding of health and social care. By 2022 more people were dying from being unable to access hospital care than were dying of Covid.

The partnership between politicians and clinicians has been developing for three-quarters of a century and has at times made the NHS one of the most admired health systems in the world in terms of accessibility, value for money, innovation, and outcomes for its patients, looking after us from 'cradle to grave'. But just as the NHS is doing poorly in the 2020s at keeping people out of the grave, we're not doing much better for those still in the cradle. In the 1960s, thanks to the NHS, the UK had the lowest neonatal mortality rate in Europe; by 1990 it had dropped into seventh place, by 2015 into nineteenth place, and five years later it had fallen a further four places to twenty-third (out of only twenty-eight countries). As former health secretary Jeremy Hunt has said, 'If the UK had the same mortality rates as Sweden, nearly 1,000 more babies would live every year.'

Back in the 1930s, when 10 per cent of all children were dead before they reached school age, the provision of medical care in Britain was dangerously uneven, and a stumbling block to the social and economic development of the country. The economist and social reformer William Beveridge famously described the obstacles to social progress as being Disease, Ignorance, Squalor, Idleness and Want. His report on approaches to tackle these obstacles, *Social Insurance and Allied Services*, was published in 1942, and intended to guide government policy for building a world beyond the Second World War. The Beveridge Report was as long as *Moby-Dick* – 200,000 words – and spelled out in dry, bureaucratic language the basic elements of a proposed welfare state. Such was the appetite in the country for social security that it became an unlikely bestseller.

In 1937 the doctor-writer A. J. Cronin, who had worked as a GP in Scotland, Wales and London, published a novel about the corruption and ineptitude of his medical colleagues. *The Citadel* spelled out in plain language the ways in which illness and poverty perpetuate one another, and just how widespread were poor standards of practice among British doctors. Part of the novel is inspired by a community in South Wales where Cronin had worked for a miners' social security cooperative – the Tredegar Medical Aid Society. Workers paid a portion of their wages into the funds of this society, and in return received medical care free of charge for themselves and their families. *The Citadel* was an international bestseller, winning a National Book Award in the United States and prompting numerous screen adaptations. Its success has often been credited with inspiring the creation of the NHS.

Aneurin Bevan was the local MP for Tredegar and later the Minister of Health in Clement Atlee's post-war Labour government. He believed in the worth of the miners' welfare fund, and that something similar should be rolled out across the country. 'Society becomes more wholesome, more serene, and spiritually healthier, if it knows that its citizens have at the back of their consciousness the knowledge that not only themselves, but all their fellows, have access, when ill, to the best that medical skill can provide', he wrote. At the time, the country's health service was a mongrel mash-up of old workhouses built under the Poor Laws, and religious and commercial institutions. 'But private charity and endowment, although inescapably essential at one time, cannot meet the cost of all this', Bevan went on. 'If the job is to be done, the state must accept financial responsibility.'

In contrast to patchy private provision, Bevan wanted a service like that enjoyed by the miners whereby everyone in the country could call upon a health professional without anxiety over their ability to pay. In place of the fear of illness there would be relief and reassurance.

In Scotland, a similar service had been set up for the Highlands and Islands region as long ago as 1913. Before state investment, this thinly populated rural area had been unable to recruit doctors and nurses. But the service guaranteed a minimum basic income to clinicians and offered support with premises and homes; thanks to the scheme there were a few decades in which rural medical care in Scotland was better than it was in the cities. Now, in the 2020s, rural communities are again suffering poorer health than those in cities by several measures: they are ageing twice as quickly as those in urban areas, and have been shown to suffer worse mental health, as well as 'diseases of despair' such as alcohol dependency. The recruitment and retention of staff in rural areas is more difficult than it is in cities.

By 1946 the British Medical Association in Scotland had agreed to cooperate in supporting a National Health Service, but many doctors in other parts of the UK were opposed. They saw the proposed NHS as a quasi-communist threat to their rights and their privileges, and were worried about becoming civil servants rather than advocates for their patients. As battles over the principles of the NHS were being fought out between Attlee's Labour government and the representatives of the medical profession, Bevan said of some hospital specialists that they 'talked about private practice as though it should be the glory of the profession. What should be the glory of the profession is that a doctor should be able to meet his patients with no financial anxiety ... we ought to take pride in the fact that, despite our financial and economic anxieties, we are still able to do the most civilised thing in the world – put the welfare of the sick in front of every other consideration.' After years of war, the UK was practically bankrupt, but in 1948 it still found the funds necessary to create the NHS.

Millions of leaflets explaining the new proposed service were distributed (I have one of them on display in my consulting room); in four concise pages each spelled out what taxpayers and the electorate would be able to expect.

> Your new National Health Service begins on 5th July. What is it? How do you get it? It will provide you with all medical, dental, and nursing care. Everyone – rich or poor, man, woman or child – can use it or any part of it. There are no charges, except for a few special items. There are no insurance qualifications. But it is not a 'charity'. You are all paying for it, mainly as taxpayers, and it will relieve your money worries in time of illness.

Readers were asked to go to the Post Office, the local library or to local council offices to pick up an application form, and to then choose a local GP to register with. 'Your dealings with your doctor will remain as they are now: *personal and confidential*. You will visit his surgery,* or he will call on you, as may be necessary. The difference is that the doctor will be paid by the Government, out of funds provided by everybody.' The new service would be 'free for all' at the point of access, but it belonged to the people, and would be funded by them.

Initially and perhaps predictably the service buckled under demand, but rather than see this as evidence that the system was unworkable, Bevan saw it as a sign of just how much unmet need there was in the country. 'Those first few years of the Service were anxious years for those of us who had the central responsibility', he wrote later. 'We were anxious, not because we feared the principles of the Service were unsound, but in case they would not be given time to justify themselves.'

Bevan had to negotiate the new NHS with

---

* In 1948 the number of female general practitioners was tiny – by 1970 it was 12 per cent, and by 1990 it was 25 per cent. Today, about 67 per cent of general practitioners are female.

doctors' representatives in the British Medical Association (BMA). General practitioners were relatively overrepresented in the BMA, and though he had many battles with them, Bevan wrote that he had a 'warm spot' for GPs, and wanted to find ways to pay them fairly without incentivising them to take on so many patients that they wouldn't be able to do their jobs properly. It's an idea that no politician has yet managed to get right.

> I was anxious to ensure that the general practitioner should be able to earn a reasonable living without having to aim at a register which would be too large to admit of good doctoring. To accomplish this I suggested a graduated system of capitation payments which would be highest in the medium ranges and lower in the higher. This would have discouraged big lists by lessening the financial inducement.

His proposal was refused – which paved the way for our current paradoxical predicament in which, for practices to survive, they are obliged to take on more and more patients until some are undoubtedly 'too large to admit of good doctoring'.

After seventy-five years of the NHS there are still no incentives or inducements for GP practices to ensure that they have manageable numbers of patients. There are no effective mechanisms to encourage continuity of care either, despite research showing that patients who are able to name their usual GP, and who are able to get a non-urgent appointment to see them, are 30 per cent less likely to access out-of-hours services overnight and at weekends, and are admitted to hospital as an emergency around 30 per cent less often. That extraordinary benefit is 'dose-dependent', so to speak, in that the longer you've been with the same GP, the better your chance of avoiding hospital or needing to use emergency services. Amazingly enough, patients who have been with the same GP for fifteen years or more have a 25 per cent lower mortality rate than people who have been registered with their practice for under a year.

If a medication could reduce your chance of hospital admission and death by a quarter we'd mandate its use, but we have a healthcare system that values prescriptions and drugs over people and time, and so policies to promote long-term relationships between doctors and their patients have been neglected. Bevan failed to have principles of continuity of care laid into the foundations of the NHS, and it's a failing that has had many consequences, among them the struggling state of GP services in today's NHS.

One side effect of the atomisation of care and the fragmentation of teams of clinicians is something one colleague of mine calls the 'Collusion of Anonymity' – when patients are handed on without anyone taking ultimate responsibility for them. Bevan worried about this when planning the NHS; as we've seen, his plan to reward GPs for keeping their list sizes manageable was rejected. One GP I know put it starkly: 'There is no reward to properly coordinate care, there's no incentive other than your own sense of professionalism to offer any continuity. For me, the best consultations build on a relationship slowly earned over dozens of encounters over many years. It's cheaper for the service and better for the patient to see someone they know.' Over a decade ago the Royal College of General Practitioners (RCGP) published a report on continuity, and concluded that 'what matters most in primary care is the quality and strength of the therapeutic relationship'. But there are still no effective mechanisms to reward continuity of care; whether or not to prioritise the strengthening of those relationships is left up to individual practices.

'There is a sound case for providing a little more money to help the doctor with a medium list who wants to make a decent living and yet be a good doctor', Bevan wrote, as if anticipating the practice closures and recruitment crises of the 2020s. 'The family doctor is in many ways the most important person in the Service.'

In the right circumstances and with the right support, the practice of medicine is enthralling both intellectually and emotionally. Performing that work within a national health service renders it even more fulfilling because clinical decisions can be made on the basis of need, rather than on the basis of ability to pay. Doctors in an NHS should be able to spend more time with patients, and less time in management meetings and poring over spreadsheets, than doctors in commercial or insurance-funded services. But political pressure to cut costs also cuts the time that each doctor or nurse has with their patient – which is why I'm often grappling with four or five significant problems in the absurdly short space of a ten-minute appointment.

For the founders of the service it was the responsibility of the community to provide all the infrastructure – hospital wards, laboratories, health centres and clinics – in which medicine could be practised, so that the profession could get on with developing high standards of care rather than developing ways of making money. Most high-income countries have a different system, topping up government spending with a mixture of insurance cover and a range of fee-for-service options. In those systems there is a basic level of healthcare for those who cannot pay, and a sliding scale of possible interventions depending on the nature of the insurance cover you're prepared to pay for, as well as a catalogue of optional treatments for those who wish to fund treatments that insurance will not cover. Those health services are as a consequence far more expensive than ours to run, but it's also worth pointing out that they're more inefficient in terms of administrative costs, with a higher proportion of health spending going into management and administration. The idea that the NHS is bloated with managers is untrue, and tends to be repeated only in sections of the media sympathetic to private interests and keen to exploit the enormous potential of healthcare to generate profit: just 2 per cent of the NHS workforce are managers, compared with around 9.5 per cent in most industries.

Because it is resourced from taxation rather than through insurance, the success of the

NHS is always going to be inextricably linked to how well it is supported by government. When government stewardship of the NHS is good it does well; when that stewardship is poor, it does badly. For too long the UK has relied on the relative efficiency of the NHS, which has very low overheads in terms of administrative costs, to justify lower spending on health than other countries. An international analysis of NHS finance and performance published in the *British Medical Journal* in 2019 concluded:

> The NHS showed pockets of good performance, including in health service outcomes, but spending, patient safety, and population health were all below average to average at best. Taken together, these results suggest that if the NHS wants to achieve comparable health outcomes at a time of growing demographic pressure, it may need to spend more to increase the supply of labour and long term care and reduce the declining trend in social spending to match levels of comparator countries.

To say that the UK cannot match the healthcare spends of France, Germany, the Netherlands or Denmark is to suggest that, as a country, the UK is too poor to have a twenty-first-century European standard of healthcare – that economically we have fallen too far behind our neighbours. Or that we have reached a point in our society where wealthy people are no longer willing to subsidise the medical care of people less fortunate. Though successive politicians have voiced frustrations with the popularity of the NHS, that very popularity has paradoxically permitted levels of underfunding and underperformance that the public wouldn't have tolerated in a service that is less well-loved.

3

THE NORMALISATION OF CRISIS: NO SLACK IN THE SYSTEM

Today's NHS: 'Crisis' headlines in the papers, protracted waiting times to see specialists, twelve-hour waits in A&E, queues of ambulances out of hospital car parks, basic drugs in short supply, a scarcity of GP appointments, operating theatres standing empty for lack of staff, queues of trolleys in corridors and, most importantly for our politicians, an unhappy electorate. Public satisfaction with the NHS is at its lowest since 1997. Doctors, nurses and paramedics have all been out on strike, and with grim regularity our hospitals overflow because of a shortage of beds and a lack of accessible social care in the community. Politicians across the political spectrum claim volubly that they adore the NHS. They lose votes when its quality drops, and gain votes when its quality improves. So why has their stewardship of it been so poor?

Since 1948 the fortunes of the NHS have shifted with the times, shuddering and cracking with tectonic movements in the political landscape. The two main political parties in the UK agree about the NHS, at least in public: they repeatedly voice support of a national health service that is mostly or entirely free at the point of delivery, in which no patient fears bankruptcy through illness, and clinicians can be free to focus on the patient, not on the patient's wallet. The Conservative Party health minister from 2012 to 2018, Jeremy Hunt, has written that 'The NHS has stood the test of time because the values it stands for have become entwined with what it means to be British.' Enoch Powell, a Conservative health minister in the early 1960s, said 'if the people have willed a National Health Service, it is because they desire it and are prepared to pay for it'. If there was ever a time when the NHS was going to be privatised, it would surely have been the 1980s, when the party of government enjoyed huge majorities and was no admirer of the founding principles of the service (although Margaret Thatcher's Conservative government did invest in the NHS more generously than have the Conservative governments of the last thirteen years). The result of more than a decade of underfunding is a system with no slack, resourced adequately only for the quietest days of summer but unable to manage demand for much of the year. It's the case now that every autumn, wards begin to overflow and trolleys stack up in corridors. To risk another plumbing metaphor: an NHS resourced adequately only for summer is a bit like having a boiler that can only keep your house warm in July.

The NHS has survived because again and again it's been shown to be deeply popular, and because the principles upon which it was founded are widely revered: that no one should fear illness because of their inability to pay for medical treatment. The sociologist T. H. Marshall memorably summarised that principle: 'Illness is neither an indulgence for which people have to pay nor an offence for which they should be penalised, but a misfortune the cost of which should be shared by the community.' The communities of this nation pay for their NHS, and they want a better service.

On 11 March 2020, as SARS-CoV2 overwhelmed the health services of better-funded, better-staffed Italy, the Chief Medical Officers of the four nations of the UK came together to write a letter to every medical practitioner in the UK. The General Medical Council, the doctors' regulator, was also a signatory. Their letter was called 'Supporting Doctors in the Event of a Covid-19 Epidemic in the UK' and was intended to reassure clinicians in GP surgeries and on hospital wards inundated by the virus that they shouldn't fear censure if they made mistakes.

How could they *not* make mistakes, when they were being asked to operate with levels of staffing, PPE, and support far below what they had been trained to expect? The letter informed all doctors in the country that 'They must bear in mind that clinicians may need to depart, possibly significantly, from established procedures in order to care for patients in the highly challenging but time-bound circumstances of the peak of an epidemic.'

It's worth lingering on that formulation 'time-bound'. Because on 14 November 2022 every clinician received a similar letter. 'The past few years have been some of the most challenging that health and social care and our professions have faced in modern times', it said. 'It's clear that there will be further challenges ahead over the coming weeks and months as we look towards winter.' As a physician I was asked to depart again from 'established procedures' not because of coronavirus, but because of annual tilting of the northern hemisphere away from the sun. The Chief Medical Officers understood that I might be fearful of making errors under the duress of winter pressures, but they would expect me to adapt my professional practice to a level appropriate to the resources available. The next few months would be 'hard going' but they would 'consider the context' in which I was working when assessing any medical negligence case made against me.

A sensible, supportive and necessary intervention of 2020, intended to reassure a workforce facing up to a frightening pandemic, had in late 2022 become something far more sinister: an acceptance of a new status quo, and a chilling normalisation of crisis.

The letter of 14 November didn't have a heading like that of March 2020, it came as a PDF by email, and its filename was simply 'Winter Regulator Letter'. The clinical workforce of the UK will likely receive another one in November 2023, and the November after that, and so on, until the chronic underfunding of the NHS is abandoned as an electoral liability, or the NHS collapses. If it does collapse it will most likely be replaced by a two-tier, insurance-funded system in which different standards of patient care will pertain for those who can pay and those who cannot, rather than the current system, in which different standards are to pertain between winter and summer. A two-tier system is essentially what we have now anyway, when so many people are paying out of their savings to get the treatment they need.

The last time I remember things being this bad was in the final years of my medical school training, in the mid-1990s, when the UK's national contribution towards health spending was just 6.3 per cent of GDP. That was in comparison to an average among the EU 14 at the time of 8.5 per cent. From the year 2000 the UK government committed to matching the EU average, and waiting lists tumbled – I can just about remember when GPs could refer a patient to a specialist clinic and expect them to be seen within twelve weeks. That all seems very long ago: since 1999 the European average spending on health has forged ahead into the double digits as a percentage of GDP, while we in the UK have fallen backwards.* After ten years of this boosted funding, the year 2010 saw public satisfaction with the NHS reach a record high. Then the government changed: a coalition was formed between the Liberal Democrats and the Conservative Party that year, and public satisfaction has fallen ever since. The number of people who are 'quite' or 'very' dissatisfied is at its highest level now for 25 years. Between 2014 and 2018, as policies of austerity began to bite, life expectancy in the UK dropped more than it did during the pandemic – a University of Oxford study ascribed that drop to cuts in health and social spending. By 2022 there were 1.6 million people on a waiting list to see a specialist about mental health, and in my area, mental health services have started sending letters out to patients saying that they won't be seen, signposting them instead to charities. It's as if we're

---

* The pandemic years were an anomaly, when huge government spending to cope with coronavirus tipped the figure temporarily higher.

returning to the patchy postcode lottery coverage of healthcare that prevailed before 1948, with charities and religious institutions taking responsibility for care.

The 'crisis' in the NHS and in its workforce has not been caused solely by Covid, or by the seasons, the Brexit-induced economic downturn, political neglect, abysmal workforce planning, the ageing population, or the rising costs of modern medical innovations, though a combination of all of these and more have hastened it. The King's Fund, a health policy advisory body, says that the NHS now needs upwards of £40 billion a year additional funds just to keep pace with our European neighbours. In 2017, the then CEO of NHS England, Simon Stevens, risked the sack when he suggested that the Brexit campaign's offer of £350 million a week to the NHS was as much a pledge to be honoured as the implementation of Brexit. But even fulfilling that promise would provide only half of what's needed.

When patients complain to me that they can't see a GP, can't walk because of their hip

pain, can't go outside because of their paralysing panic attacks, can't sleep for the torment
of a skin condition, or that they're struggling
with disabling bladder or bowel problems, I try
not to become despondent about the steady
diminution of adequate resourcing, or angry
that they can't access the specialist care I think
they need. Instead I try to comfort myself with
the quietly radical idea that at some level, this
must be the level of NHS funding that the UK
government thinks the people will tolerate,
and that they voted for. But it's not the government's service, it's ours, and if we want a
higher-quality service with shorter waiting
times, we have to insist on it at the ballot box.

Many of my colleagues are convinced that
the NHS needs to be unhitched from political cycles; that it's too easily blown off course
by the winds of political change; that it needs
a cross-party board that would oversee the
service with a timeframe and a depth of vision
beyond the lifetimes of parliaments. I hold
sympathy with that view, but am also anxious
that such a cross-party body would be blamed

for NHS failures that have their roots in under-funding rather than in poor management. As an electorate we would lose the ability to register our displeasure with the government of the country when the NHS is being failed.

Before the pandemic our hospitals were under-resourced and overwhelmed. We already have among the lowest hospital bed numbers in Europe, and safe limits are breached routinely, not only in winter. Former NHS England chief Simon Stevens said as long ago as 2017 that the NHS was no longer funded adequately to cope with what was being asked of it. A year earlier Stevens had warned presciently that 'if general practice fails, the whole NHS fails'. By 2019 a friend who is a consultant geriatrician told me how her hospital was obliged to pack five patients into bays designed only for four – that's five patients sharing one toilet, four sets of curtains for privacy, four oxygen outlets, and, more crucially, nurses sufficient for the care of only four patients. Two patients had been squeezed into a room designed for carrying out endoscopies, with no curtains for patient privacy and no bathroom. Four-bedded bays now routinely house *six* in winter, and they're the lucky ones who manage to get a bed rather than a trolley in a corridor. Staffing levels that even three or four years ago would have been considered unacceptably risky have become routine. Outpatient clinics for several specialties have waiting lists so long that they might as well not exist. In my area, at the time of writing, urgent colorectal surgery referrals have a waiting time of fifty-seven weeks; dermatology appointments take ninety-one weeks.

This is a service that's no longer a service, a level of overwhelm that piles ever more pressure back into the community as patients are told: the hospitals are full, see your GP instead. 'If general practice fails, the whole NHS fails' was a warning that went unheeded; in the winter of 2022–23 A&E waiting times and GP access figures showed that the two front-facing specialties of the NHS, general practice and emergency medicine, were in free fall. The vice chair of the Royal College of Emergency Medicine in Scotland, Dr Fiona Hunter, said in an interview with the BBC: 'I never want to work another winter like that, and I don't want the patients to have to go through another winter like that within urgent care. There are patients at risk within the emergency department and throughout the hospital.' She was particularly anxious about the demoralising effect of such underfunding on staff: 'We need to stop staff leaving in their droves, make our staff feel valued, allow them to come to work and do a caring job and leave the shift feeling that they've made a difference.' The outlook, she said, was 'bleak'. The palliative care doctor and writer Rachel Clarke put it more starkly:

> I am angry with every molecule of my being because I am going to work and literally seeing patients dying on trolleys who did not have to die and would not have died if the government and the party in power for the last thirteen years had made different political choices. These deaths are not

the way the world is. These are daily avoidable deaths as a result of political choices
that the government of the day doesn't
even have the integrity to acknowledge.
And instead all they do is turn their faces
from the dying and deny that there's a crisis
at all.

Towards the close of last winter a BBC
journalist interviewed Amanda McCabe, a consultant paediatric surgeon, who said of staffing:
'There is a huge amount of goodwill in the
NHS and it's important that this isn't eroded by
the pressures being put on healthcare workers.
Steps must be taken to ensure NHS staff are
valued, nurtured, and supported.' This crisis
in workforce morale and retention is the most
pressing of the many difficulties the NHS is now
suffering as a consequence of sustained political
neglect. The interviewee representing general
practice recounted similarly unbearable pressures on the system – something borne out by
my own experience. Practices all around my
own are being forced to close their lists to new

patients, and some are closing their doors altogether, telling the local health board that they can't go on. Around eight hundred UK practices have closed their doors in the last ten years.

Here are some examples from last winter. An elderly patient of mine spent more than twenty-four hours on a corridor trolley before a bed could be found. Another patient with chronic inflammatory bowel disease, a condition that can lead to sepsis and bowel perforation, developed an agonising abdominal pain. He went, appropriately, to A&E, where he sat on a hard chair for seven hours before being admitted by harried, exhausted-looking staff. The ward was, he said, 'bedlam' and after forty-eight hours he was discharged with contradictory letters describing his stay, and no improvement in his pain. I spent much of a morning when I should have been seeing the fourteen patients on my clinic list trying to manage what should have been addressed in hospital. Later in the week I called an ambulance for a frail vulnerable woman who'd fallen down a flight of stairs and snapped her wrist.

Her hand was very swollen, the blood flow sluggish, meaning that she needed her wrist to be straightened urgently – but the call handler told me to expect an ambulance to take four or maybe five hours. One paramedic told me that in the course of a twelve-hour shift he had managed to take only two patients to hospital – not for lack of calls, but because ten of those hours were spent in queues outside A&E unable to offload his patients. It's now normal for people with problems that require hospital admission to present to general practice instead because they're terrified of the chaos of A&E, and in the past few months several frail elderly patients have pleaded with me not to send them in. The pandemic mantra of 'Protect the NHS' hasn't helped – some people are so reluctant to avoid being a burden on the system that they're staying away, when it could be argued that the purpose of the NHS is to protect *them*. Medicine is supposed to ease suffering, but inadequate resources mean that suffering is being amplified and extended by failures of the NHS to meet demand.

My profession of general practice has become punch-drunk from successive waves of reform, inadequate staff numbers, and the insistence that it take over management of almost all chronic disease that occurs in a population that's older and frailer than it has ever been, as well as address the ballooning mental health needs of a society traumatised by the ordeal of the pandemic (and one increasingly encouraged to seek out mental health support) – all without an expansion of the workforce or real-terms resource. *That* is why people are struggling to get an appointment, not because of inefficiency or because doctors are workshy. As calls go out to 'name and shame' practices reeling from these blows, GPs are providing more appointments than they were before the pandemic. But even those improved levels of availability have been overtaken by demand, and many practices feel that they can't revert to normal, face-to-face consulting because they can only just cope with demand if they try phoning every patient first, to see if the problem can be addressed at a distance. A rule of medical training is 'always see the patient' – if you haven't put a hand on their painful belly or a stethoscope on their wheezing chest or peered into their aching throat then you haven't properly assessed the patient, but many doctors are so pressed by demand that they feel it impossible to return to full face-to-face clinics.

As the population ages, and recovers from the trauma of the pandemic, the demands from patients have risen steadily, but the funds made available by the taxpayer are not keeping pace with what is expected by those same taxpayers. The result is a drop in professional standards across the service, and leads to a vicious cycle: specialists in hospitals can't meet their own demand, and so seek to transfer more and more of what they used to do onto GPs in the community. GPs can't meet their own demand, and so it becomes impossible to get an appointment, and people turn up in unprecedented numbers in A&E. Now, with the most senior government health advisers in the UK, the Chief Medical Officers, expecting care standards to deteriorate with the annual change of the seasons, we can see that something fundamental has shifted in the foundations of my profession. The result is a new mode of practising medicine that is less about quality of care than it is about surviving, less about healing than it is about damage limitation.

As I write, in the summer of 2023, the NHS is looking towards autumn and another winter. There's no slack in the system right now, no spare bed capacity, no new doctors or new nurses waiting in the wings – so how will it cope as sickness rates rise with the slide into winter? The worry is that we will have even fewer staff this year than last because of industrial disputes and low morale from having to fight every day to help patients get through a failing system. As NHS workers, our summers are now spent bracing ourselves for winter. We're barely into the autumn when patients start pleading not to be sent in to hospital.

To be in crisis used to mean being at the mercy of the subtlest of interventions, any of which might prove decisive in tipping the patient towards recovery or demise. Winter 'crises' have been declared so many times that the phrase has been drained of any sense of drama. The gravity of the service's problems are different this time: like a patient on life support, the NHS hangs in the balance, at the mercy of our politicians and of us, as an electorate. There's still time to save it, but if I had to break the news to loved ones, I'd say it's touch and go whether it will pull through.

4

WORKFORCE: WE'RE ALL ON THE SAME TEAM

Healthcare is people work, and it needs to be done by people. A system that still runs on 1990s computing power and pagers is unlikely to be replaced by robots or algorithms any time soon. AI algorithms don't work very well in healthcare anyway – they don't engage with people's need for *care*, and they are programmed to have a tolerance for risk so low that, in my experience, they often send people to hospital or to their NHS GP urgently for investigations of symptoms that simply need a human conversation, and reassurance. A system that will send almost anyone with a headache for a brain scan and almost anyone with a twinge in their breastbone to A&E to have their heart checked is unlikely to cost the taxpayer less than the system we have now.

We don't have enough nurses, doctors and allied health professionals to manage all the health conversations that the population needs or expects. It's becoming more apparent that the country's traditional approach to these shortages – import trained professionals from abroad – is no longer working, in part because of concerns over exacerbating a brain drain from other countries, and in part because the UK is steadily becoming a less attractive destination for overseas professionals. Training programmes are belatedly increasing capacity, and it will take a few years for healthier numbers of trained clinicians to come through. Bursaries for medical and nursing students from modest backgrounds would help, with admissions procedures that take account of the significant barriers students from deprived communities face. In 1971 a GP called Julian Tudor Hart wrote of what he called the 'inverse

care law': 'The availability of good medical
care tends to vary inversely with the need for it
in the population served. This inverse care law
operates more completely where medical care
is most exposed to market forces, and less so
where such exposure is reduced.' Tudor Hart
noted the blatant inequities that market forces
introduce into healthcare: 'the market distribu-
tion of healthcare is a primitive and outdated
social form, and any return to it would further
exaggerate the maldistribution of medical
resources.'

Medical students who grew up in communities of relative social deprivation have been
shown to be far more likely than wealthier
peers to want to work in the kinds of areas
and communities where they grew up. Any
initiatives to encourage school students from
modest backgrounds into healthcare should
be better supported. One of my colleagues
also insists that the introduction of university
fees for healthcare courses has been a disaster:
clinicians who have been trained by the taxpayer feel a great deal more loyalty and sense

of service than people who've been obliged to pay for their university education themselves.

An unhappy consequence of the squeeze on NHS resources over the past few years is a noticeable diminution of fellow feeling between colleagues who, in an attempt to manage their own patients to a high standard, are increasingly obliged to reject requests for help or advice. As already mentioned, psychiatry is now so under-resourced that GP referrals are routinely rejected without explanation, and even those patients whose referrals are accepted can wait four or five years. This leads to a lottery of care in which some conditions continue to be managed to exemplary, world-class standards, while others are utterly neglected. Urgent and cancer care trumps everything else, so chronic conditions get pushed further and further to the back of the to-do list, or their referrals simply refused, referrals handed back to referrers. Doctors and nurses are accustomed to viewing themselves as members of a team – a competitive mindset is alien to both their training and their thinking – but as resources diminish, and

demand rises, clinicians are asked to see themselves as competitors, squabbling on behalf of
their patients over the few scraps of funding
that fall their way.

The joys of working in the NHS are many:
the pleasure of helping patients, the variety
and interest of the work, the intellectual challenges, the emotional rewards, the satisfactions
of being part of a team that, for some specialties, is countrywide. I worked once in India,
and remember taking over responsibility for
a patient with a rare, complex lung disease,
whose problems went beyond my expertise. I
asked a colleague who I could refer to for advice:
'Do you have any friends who are pulmonolo-
gists?' he replied, 'isn't there anyone you could
phone?' At that hospital there was no hierarchy
of specialists available to offer reliable advice,
so my patient's health would depend on my
chance networks of acquaintance.

By contrast, as a GP in the NHS I can call
up just about any clinician in the country,
Derry to Dover, Lerwick to Lyme Regis, and
if we have a patient in common, we will help

one another. At the local level too, NHS clinicians come together daily with the same aim: physicians, dieticians, physiotherapists, social workers, psychiatrists, speech and language and occupational therapists, not to mention all the non-clinical staff who keep the wheels of clinics and hospitals turning. Until relatively recently it felt like a privilege to be part of a system so cherished for its principles. Most workers in the NHS felt they had gained personally and professionally by working for such a valued organisation, and they were happy to feel as if they were giving something back to their communities.

After a decade's squeeze on funding that feeling is much rarer now. Prior to the pandemic the system was under immense strain – the consequence of nine years of underfunding, as well as near-zero capital investment, and stagnating wages. Real-term pay as well as working conditions had steadily deteriorated. On the eve of the pandemic, the Royal College of Nursing estimated that the UK was short of 43,000 nurses. Six in every ten nurses felt that they weren't able to do their jobs properly because of staff shortages. In 2022, nurses were being paid a fifth less than they had been a decade earlier, and many were leaving the profession for jobs where they'd earn better pay, their skills would be better appreciated, and they would have better opportunities to look after their own mental health. I know of acute medical wards where, because of staff absence, there is often only one nurse covering an *entire ward* – no wonder my patient Helen R. was able to fall unnoticed and break her hip.

Recently, I spoke with a community occupational therapist who told me that her own team, whose work is critical in getting people safely back home from hospital, is supposed to have four members of staff, but three posts are unfilled – she has to work alone. Midwives too are in short supply – the Royal College of Midwives reports that we have 2,500 fewer of them than are needed. Another ward I know of recently lost almost all its clinical support workers because a coffee chain nearby was offering better pay. The stress of the pandemic led to an exhausted and overwhelmed workforce; and in the space of just a few months patients have gone from offering spontaneous expressions of love for the NHS, clapping healthcare workers from their doorsteps, to cursing and criticising the same people for service failures that have their origins in political decisions, not clinical ones. The suicide risk for healthcare workers is 24 per cent higher than the national average – a shocking figure largely explained by the number of young female nurses who die by suicide. But doctors also have higher suicide rates than average – particularly doctors who have been the subject of patient complaints, which are also on the rise.

The figures for newly qualified doctors leaving the UK or even leaving the profession are no less worrying. Doctors are called 'junior' until they complete speciality training, which can take ten or fifteen years. These highly qualified professionals now rarely work as part of a defined clinical team, and frequently struggle to develop mentor relationships with their seniors, because there are vanishingly few opportunities to learn along-side someone much more experienced. Many parts of the NHS are so stressed that anyone with minimal training is expected to work independently, with little protected time in the day to talk, reflect and share responsibility with seniors. That level of unsupported responsibility is frightening for the junior doctors and unsafe for the patient; the statistics for how many newly qualified doctors are now leaving programmes of UK training to plug gaps else-where in the world (mostly Australia) were described to me by one consultant colleague as truly shocking. 'We're getting something very, very wrong with training,' she said to me, 'or we're training the wrong people. Our juniors are hugely unhappy in the main. We're struggling with retention and recruitment.' Another told me that current training is far too rigid. 'Going off to do other things is seen as too negative. We don't embrace that these juniors are talented, capable individuals. And we teach them that all that matters is that they do all these tick-box clinical competencies. We stifle them, treat them as infants, we call them juniors until they're about forty!' One consultant echoed my GP colleague, telling me that the introduction of university fees had been one of the most salient reasons for a change in morale among the new generation of doctors: 'They've paid through the nose to get here, and then they're exploited. Why should they have any love for the NHS? But my own generation felt grateful for their education, which was paid for by the taxpayer, and felt as if they had an obligation to give something back. They felt grateful for their job, and felt much more valued.'

The pandemic saw healthcare workers everywhere in the world obliged to work for many months through appalling conditions, often in overwhelmed wards – all without adequate protective equipment and little compensation. Students as young as third years were expected to take on responsible roles, even communicating between family members and patients dying of Covid. In the UK at least, clinicians saw lockdown rules disregarded by the very people who made them. But we *did* receive some compensation: when the dust began to settle, my own local area supplied every health worker with an A5 rainbow certificate and a small metal badge. Finishing a shift at the GP out-of-hours centre at the local hospital one night I saw a pile of them in the bin.

Through 2022, as the world began to gently emerge into a post-pandemic reality, the NHS was in a sad and depleted state, its already inadequate workforce even less able to cope. Then began the onslaught: the delayed presentations of serious disease, the surge of demand as the backed-up problems and pent-up misery of two years of lockdowns came crashing back through GP surgeries and A&E – the front doors of the NHS – precipitating the most savage winter crisis I've yet seen, that of 2022–23. A demoralised NHS workforce woke up to a surging workload but nothing to look forward to in terms of new initiatives, new streams of funding, better pay or more joined-up thinking on patient flow through the service. They were asked simply to keep doing more with less. Widespread strikes among nurses, junior doctors and paramedics were the result.

In the past, NHS workers got on with the difficulties of their jobs because they felt they were making a difference to patients' lives and they still felt valued by the organisation and by their colleagues. What we're seeing now is a crisis in morale that has tangled roots in decades of negligent workforce planning and exacerbated by a frail ageing population, rising patient expectations, and diminishing resources with which to manage them. 'The system compensated, and compensated, and compensated,' one senior clinician told me, 'and then suddenly the stress of the pandemic flipped it into a new paradigm.' He explained how funding, morale, public support and staff- ·ing all began to drain away, and widespread disenchantment and disappointment among those left began to grow. 'It's as if those with political responsibility for the NHS would like to see it undermined,' he added, remind- ing me of a line of Aneurin Bevan's about the

Conservative Party of the 1950s: 'If the Service could be killed they wouldn't mind, but they would wish it done more stealthily and in such a fashion that they would not appear to have responsibility.'

Stamina and capacity to take on new streams of work are both at a low point. Failing services are unhappy places to work, and people vote with their feet, nudging those services further into a downwards spiral. There are over 110,000 unfilled posts within NHS England, and in my own area, advertisements for consultant and GP positions regularly return no applicants. 'More staff would make a huge difference,' one specialist trainee doctor told me 'because everyone would have less pressure, fewer patients, and more time to do their job well, and to *feel* they're doing their job well. None of us currently do. We feel undervalued. We are just there to plug a service gap and see people on continual ward rounds. And the same goes for the nurses.'

Lack of admin support means that consultants are spending large parts of their day on typing and secretarial tasks with outdated computer systems, at a time when administrative workload is increasing. 'I get lots of emails about signing off results, or that I haven't "outcomed" my clinic patients on the system,' one consultant told me, 'but no one is looking at whether I'm caring for my patients. It's process over care.'

What can be done? No one is denying that the service is currently under-resourced for what is being asked of it, and so if no more new money and staff are forthcoming it's necessary to start a national conversation about what the NHS can continue to do, and what it will have to stop doing. As the President of the Royal College of Physicians in Edinburgh put it recently: 'Can we really afford to provide everything that is available, for everybody, across their entire life course? And if we cannot, how should we decide what we can provide? Although politicians will have views, and doctors can advise, the public must have a say.' Workforce morale would undoubtedly improve with better pay (full-time specialist registrars have seen the value of their wages drop by 20 per cent since 2010), but that's not enough on its own – as one colleague who works as a cancer specialist said to me, 'the half-life of satisfaction with more pay is short, and there are plenty of unhappy doctors with a thriving private practice'. What's needed are new ways of promoting team working, a shared sense of purpose, the opportunity to work together rather than in isolation.

Medical care has become fragmented, with the atomisation of roles and a dilution of the sense of individual responsibility for the patient. Each hospital and primary care trust needs to make time and money available for new ways of fostering re-enchantment with the ideals and principles and satisfactions of what has always been challenging but rewarding work. If they do not, staffing problems will only get worse.

The new generation of young doctors look at the workload of their seniors, at the attrition of their pay, at the conditions, and quite understandably conclude 'I'm not doing that'.

'All my juniors hate their job' one consultant told me in despair. 'At their stage I loved mine. There's been a huge attitude shift – in my day I did always have to work late, but I felt that I was doing a good job. Now the juniors have reached the point that, since they know the work can never done, and since they're only paid until 5 p.m., they announce "I'm going home", even though there are patients that still need to be seen. They have a point, but it doesn't help your working environment and it doesn't help the team.'

New models of working need to be developed that accept a mix of patient-facing, teaching, and research time as a standard part of the working week for clinicians across the service. 'Huge numbers of trainees are asking to work less than full time,' one training director told me. 'Which is a marker of changing times, but also reflects the juniors' unhappiness with the hours and the conditions in which they are working. They expect a more varied career, which is a good thing. But when someone moves to three days per week, and personally takes that pay cut, the hospital's saving on their salary can't be allocated to someone else. That needs to change because it leaves the service short, and would be so easy to fix.' At the moment general practice is different: if someone takes less pay for working fewer hours, the saving *can* be used to pay other doctors. It wouldn't be too difficult for hospitals to do the same.

One colleague told me that she'd like to see clinicians grouped back into named teams with responsibility for a defined group of patients, though another warned me that the old team-based approach could be awful 'if your face didn't fit'. Another said: 'Spend a little on keeping your staff happy and that would help', and wanted to see hospital social events encouraged and supported. One GP told me that during his own junior training there was a 7.30 a.m. handover every morning in a hospital mess-room, with coffee and breakfast rolls provided. That tiny catering cost to the hospital more than paid for itself in better staff morale and vastly improved patient care: the outgoing night staff would talk with the incoming day staff about the problems of the night, the patients who were a worry, the challenges the day might bring – and, crucially, everyone in the meeting had the opportunity to feel that they were playing a part in something bigger than themselves, and were developing a sense of a shared mission. 'That's all gone now,' another told me when I relayed this story; 'handovers are just emailed Word documents on a screen.'

Managers need to acknowledge that many staff are exhausted beyond what might be remedied by mindfulness sessions or debriefing chats over a sandwich. For many years now clinicians have been patching together the service, and are worn out by the extra effort of trying to do the right thing by their patients as well as the emotional labour of always having to apologise for NHS failings. 'It's death by a thousand cuts,' a consultant surgeon said to me. 'The current climate is a symptom of the dysfunction that's been building for years, and is now everywhere in the service.'

For some colleagues I interviewed while

researching this book the priority of NHS managers should be to stall the general slide towards specialism, and reverse the growing lack of respect for generalism. Training programmes of the future might need to spend more time and space exploring what it means to be a 'good enough' generalist doctor, able to manage the majority of conditions in their remit, though able to recognise when someone might benefit from a more specialist perspective. 'We used to do this,' one despondent general physician told me, 'but it wasn't supported, wasn't respected, and now it'll take a decade to get back to what we had.' At consultant level there is still a great deal of siloed thinking; 'cardiology, gastrointestinal medicine, respiratory, they are losing the ability to look after frail complicated patients,' one geriatrician told me. 'And my own speciality isn't big enough to take everything on.' The GP Phil Whitaker, in his book *What is a Doctor?*, put it like this: 'When someone becomes unwell, the earlier they encounter an experienced medical generalist to make a biopsychosocial diagnosis, the more appropriate and holistic their care, and the more cost-effective for the NHS as a whole. Disrupt this generalist layer in the NHS and increasing numbers of patients are sucked inappropriately into resource-intensive emergency and specialist services.' If our politicians don't want to invest in generalism, but wish instead to prioritise access to specialists, the evidence is plain: the NHS is going to need a *lot* more money.

The NHS is immense (imagine a healthcare body so large that can be short of 43,000 nurses and still function at all), and reforms are very slow to take effect, but incremental changes in training are now encouraging consultants to be generalists with special interests. One of the consultants I interviewed told me that 'there's a lot to be hopeful for, and there's no other job that I would do. Whether you want to fix people, or simply help them, whether you want to use your hands or your brain, I can't think of any profession that is as varied as medicine, and at the end of the day it gives me a massive kick when I get a good outcome for a patient.' Another told me: 'A state of the art health service needs adequate funding. Are we a rich country or a poor one? If we're a relatively rich one, why don't we have a health service to match?'

5

PATIENTS OR SHAREHOLDERS? THE REALITIES OF COMMERCIAL MEDICINE

A few years ago I was asked if I'd consider working in a private GP clinic – one of those city-centre enterprises with a sleek logo, an expensive address, and an eye on the wallets of bankers. The word 'private' as used in healthcare is oddly misleading – these services are no more confidential than NHS services, and they should more properly be called 'commercial', in that they sell clinical services on a commercial basis. I had a part-time job in the NHS at the time, and was looking for a bit of extra work: I wondered if the clinic would be a rewarding place to do it. At their invitation I went for a look around. The convenience of its location was indisputable, its decor was immaculate, and its clinical standards, I was assured, were irreproachable. Towards the end of my tour I asked one of the GPs about their procedure for writing private prescriptions.

The cost of a drug is set by the pharmaceutical company that developed it, for as long as they hold the patent (usually twenty years). After the patent has expired any drug manufacturer can make and sell a 'generic' version of the drug, and the costs become subject to market forces. The price of drugs, both for the patient and to the taxpayer, influences the way that doctors prescribe. Study after study has shown that NHS GPs are not just conscious of drug costs but that they attempt to reduce those costs through a variety of strategies, and do so without compromising the effectiveness of the care they provide. I was interested in the clinic's attitude to prescriptions because private medicine is different – some doctors in the sector have even been known to prescribe expensive drugs, in the belief that patients will have more faith in them when they are paying (and also that if a drug costs just pennies it can't be any good). The response to my enquiry surprised me: 'Patients pay the full price of whatever they're prescribed,' he said, 'but we also have an arrangement with a pharmacy around the corner. They charge a private dispensing fee on top of the cost of the drug, and part of that fee makes its way back to us for giving them the business.' Surprise must have shown on my face because he shrugged, and became defensive. 'It's all perfectly legal,' he went on, 'we're providing a service, and patients are happy to pay.'

In the Middle Ages physicians justified their appetite for gold by using it as a constituent of expensive medication regimes (it's still there in the formulary today, listed between 'goitre' and 'golfer's elbow', as an intramuscular injection to ease rheumatoid arthritis). When Bevan was asked how he'd overcome the resistance of hospital consultants to his new National Health Service, he'd allegedly said that he'd 'stuffed their mouths with gold'. In getting specialists' agreement, Bevan was obliged to leave the door open for them to splice commercial work with NHS work, a concession that fifty years later, when working as a junior hospital doctor, I witnessed causing problems both for patients and for NHS staff. When I started training in the 1990s some consultants couldn't be contacted when doing their private work even at the time they were supposed to be on call for the NHS. I even worked with one who brought her private patients in to have operations in the NHS hospital at the weekend. This could have dramatic repercussions not just on staff workload, but for NHS patients: I remember one private patient, brought in for weekend surgery because of the inadequate facilities at the local private hospital, becoming so unwell post-operatively that I had to spend most of my weekend on call at her bedside, attending to her soaring fevers and crashing blood pressure. At that time NHS patients who were likely to become unwell after complex surgery had their operations early in the week so that their immediate post-op care would, for several days, be in a fully staffed ward. This private patient needed so much medical attention over a thinly staffed weekend that the needs of all the other patients on the ward were neglected, and the good will and professionalism of NHS staff was exploited.

In my work as an NHS GP the corrupting effect of commercial and private medicine is less immediately obvious, but through my correspondence with specialists I know that it still goes on: scans, arthroscopies and follow-up appointments are all more lavishly recommended when the patient is paying, which makes one wonder about the criteria used to recommend them. Operations are more lavishly recommended too. I remember an angry father who insisted I refer his son for a tonsillectomy after a couple of episodes of tonsillitis. If I want to refer someone to have their tonsils out on the NHS, the local surgeons won't countenance seeing them unless they meet certain criteria: seven episodes of tonsillitis in the last year, or ten over the last two years, or three a year for the last three consecutive years. There are good reasons for this: tonsillectomy risks haemorrhage and infection, as well as leaving you more prone to throat problems in the future. Though we all pay for NHS care through taxation, no doctor in the NHS will now remove your tonsils just because you've asked them to – that would be considered a grave abandonment of professional standards, and a flouting of evidence-based practice. But the private healthcare market specialises in commercial treatment on demand, and the rules are different over there. When the father repeated his demand at a private clinic the surgeon's professional reservations melted away: the operation was scheduled within days. The surgeon's clinic letter contained within it a tortured justification for tabling the surgery that was painful to read. It must have been painful, too, for the patient, who went on to need NHS hospital admission to address subsequent complications (bleeding, infection). Several of my own clinic appointments were used to deal with the aftermath. There is as yet no reliable mechanism for the NHS to bill private health companies for the expenses incurred when private procedures go wrong. Andrew Lees, a professor of neurology in London, has written of private healthcare: 'Private hospitals are there to generate income and all the rhetoric of quality, safety and patient satisfaction is in truth no more than a public relations exercise.' Of his colleagues who work in private practice, Lees has observed that they are obliged to be 'factory workers in what has become a service industry. Their efforts to be kind and treat the patient as an individual are stymied at every stage by an enterprise culture that follows the money.'

A patient of mine once went to a private oncologist for chemotherapy – an unusual choice, given that cancer services have generally been the most protected from NHS underfunding. I was surprised when late one afternoon he called me to ask for an NHS prescription of broad spectrum antibiotics. The private oncologist had called him to say that his blood tests had shown a low white cell count as a consequence of chemotherapy. White blood cells fight infection, so a low count put my patient at risk of sepsis. NHS protocols for the management of low white counts are strict, and recommend antibiotics only in the case of a fever, and after numerous further blood tests have been carried out. So for me to issue the prescription would have been to abandon standard protocols. I suspected that this was for the convenience of the oncologist, not for the benefit of the patient, and tried to get in touch with the oncologist. When I finally managed to track him down he was on a Mediterranean beach, and admitted that the patient had only been redirected to me for such unorthodox treatment because he was out of the country.

Private providers sell an image of excellence and efficiency, but that glossy sheen, in the UK at least, is built on the assurance that whenever a patient becomes unprofitable, or presents too much of a risk, the NHS will step in. Following the 2012 NHS reforms brought in by the Coalition government's Minister for

Health, Andrew Lansley, it was predicted that private companies would engage in a free-for-all over aspects of NHS services. But ten years on we can see that that didn't happen: many of the companies who won supposedly lucrative contracts within the NHS have long since handed them back because of low profitability, or because they'd been offering worryingly low standards of care. Lansley's 2012 Health and Social Care Act was finally torn up and discarded in the 2022 Health and Care Act, when it was quietly acknowledged that in-house NHS services are significantly more efficient for the taxpayer than contracting out to private companies.

Over the last forty years a model of profit and competition has become embedded in the way society thinks about public services; even to challenge that model has begun to seem naive. Privatisation hasn't worked for the railways, which are gradually sliding back into public hands, and it didn't work for health services either. Privatised and commercially-driven health services are more fragmented, more transactional, less holistic, more socially divisive and unjust, and provide ultimately poorer care (for evidence, look at the health outcomes of the US, which are the worst in the developed world). The NHS is one of the few corners of our society in which a privatising model has been repeatedly rejected, but some lobby groups continue to advocate for it against all the evidence.

One afternoon a couple of years ago my clinic was interrupted by a phone call from a concerned psychologist who worked for a large private health company. It's not unusual for patients who have enough money to pay for a private psychologist or counsellor in addition to seeing an NHS psychiatrist, because NHS mental health services are so threadbare. It's frustrating to work within a service that is so under-resourced, but I'm often glad when a patient can afford additional mental health support. The psychologist had insisted to the receptionist that she speak with me immediately, because she had grave concerns about one of my patients – let's call him Walter. 'Walter's here with me,' she said from her office with an expensive address, 'and he's desperately suicidal.'

'Bring him over,' I said, 'I'll fit him in.'

When I went to call Walter from the waiting room he was alone – the psychologist hadn't waited to tell me more about her concerns. 'I've no idea why I'm here,' he said as he took a seat in my office, almost embarrassed. 'I don't feel any different today than usual.' It took a while to unpick the sequence of events: he'd told the psychologist that he often felt low and had, in the past, contemplated suicide. But he currently had no active plans to kill himself. He'd been seen by one of my GP colleagues only the week before and had follow-up appointments arranged with ourselves as well as with the NHS psychiatrists the following week (none of which the psychologist had asked him about). He was bewildered by having been spirited over to my waiting room then abandoned by a private healthcare system confident that the NHS would take over as soon as he might present a risk.

The former health secretary Jeremy Hunt was well aware that tendering out NHS services to private companies can have profoundly detrimental effect on the NHS as a whole. He wrote of the paradox: 'independent hospitals fish from the same pool of doctors for their workforce – indeed, they employ NHS doctors for much of their work. Over-reliance on the private sector therefore sucks doctors and nurses out of NHS hospitals, making waiting lists even longer.' Private medical companies benefit by using specialists who are trained and have their professional standards maintained through another body – the NHS. They can, at times, use NHS facilities and NHS staff to care for their sickest patients, when their own facilities are not up to standard, which happens often. As an example, in my own city local surgeons complain that the main private hospital doesn't have a high-quality operating microscope, obliging them to use NHS facilities. Professional standards of evidence-based practice are flouted in the private sector, because treatment is often offered on demand rather than according to best evidence. Prices in the private sector are kept artificially low because, in the UK at least, private providers can avoid paying for the fallout of their mistakes – NHS colleagues will follow up any infections and bleeds post-operatively, and if everything goes wrong you can always phone an NHS ambulance (if you suffer a heart attack in many small private hospitals, they phone 999). These factors all mean that private companies can afford to sell an image of efficiency and modernity that in truth they have little claim on, because their success is predicated on the existence of the NHS. They also benefit from a failing NHS, because more and more people have to dip into savings to get the treatment they need.

There is, however, another means by which private companies profit from the existence of the NHS: the use or abuse of clinical records. NHS medical records, meticulously gathered over decades for the benefit of the patient, provide a tremendous resource to mine for risk stratification, enabling private insurers to optimise their own profit margins – they can gain access to these with the signed agreement of the patient. I once had a long-running correspondence with an insurance company about a patient of mine who had varicose vein surgery privately, rather than wait for it on the NHS. A company representative had trawled through her NHS notes and insisted that a historical reference to leg pain proved that the patient had lied about the exact year her varicose veins began to trouble her. If I would only agree that the 'leg pain' entry in her notes represented an early sign of varicose veins, then it would qualify as a 'pre-existing condition' and the costs of her vein surgery could be demanded back from the patient. When I argued that the notes said no such thing, and that the earliest moment when diagnosis becomes possible is often a grey area, I was told that 'we work with liabilities, there are no grey areas'. It was starkly obvious that the company's ultimate duty was to its shareholders, while my own duty, under the auspices of the NHS, was to act in the interests of the patient sitting before me.

Health is like power, education or money – it confers social advantage according to how much of it you have in comparison to others. In a society that's increasingly unequal private health companies are booming, while we're told a 'free NHS' is unaffordable. The NHS isn't really free – we all pay for it through our taxes, and we'll get the service we are willing to pay for.

I have many colleagues who have worked in the Republic of Ireland, in Australia and in New Zealand, where mandatory insurance, direct payments and co-payments make up a substantial portion of the way services are funded. Up to a third of junior doctors today are leaving UK training schemes to work in these countries because pay and conditions in Britain are now so poor by comparison. GMC figures report that there are 18,000 UK-trained doctors practising overseas – a number that has gone up by 50 per cent since 2008. In another GMC survey, doctors leaving the NHS were asked their reason for leaving the UK: 35.7 per cent reported 'dissatisfaction with role, place of work, NHS culture' and 27.2 per cent reported 'burnout and work-related stress'.

Among clinicians I've spoken to who have gone to work elsewhere, without exception they prefer the *system* of the NHS, when it works, because of the way it encourages treatment on the basis of need rather than demand. But one consultant told me this year that for the first time in her career she has started to consider working in private healthcare. 'It has recently occurred to me that the NHS might just fall apart,' she said, 'and increasingly it's looking as if the only way to offer effective care might be in the private sector, where I could set my own standards. That shows how worried I am that the NHS is failing, and offering poorer standards than I'm comfortable with.' She wondered whether it might be wise to look into how to set herself up as a commercial provider of healthcare. 'But at the same time I feel very much defined by my profession and very committed to the NHS.'

In the end I decided against working in that

private clinic: too many aspects of the place made me uneasy. The arrangement they had between themselves and a local pharmacy struck me as a new manifestation of an old alliance: doctors and apothecaries have a long and dishonourable tradition of joining forces to supplement their incomes. The practice was already ancient seven hundred years ago, when Chaucer mocked a physician for it in his Prologue to the *Canterbury Tales:*

> Prepared he was, with his apothecaries,
> To send him drugs and electuaries;
> By mutual aid much gold they'd always
>   won –
> Their friendship was a thing not new
>   begun

In Old Scots the word *avareis* or 'avarice' has two meanings: the usual sense of 'greed', evolved from the Latin *avarus*, but also 'a duty or impost on goods; a charge additional to the freight'. There were several reasons I didn't want to work in the private clinic, but the 'avareis' charge arranged between them and their apothecaries was a prominent one. I wondered how many other aspects of their practice might be skewed in favour of income generation, rather than the best interests of the patient.

We've been here before, and long before Chaucer: more than two thousand years ago the authors known collectively as 'Hippocrates' were clear on the subject of how money affects clinical practice: it corrupts. As the NHS is denigrated by those in power, and private medicine is promoted as an example of efficiency and consumer-friendliness, it's worth remembering some of them. 'One must not be anxious about fixing a fee,' Hippocrates says in the *Precepts*. 'For I consider such a worry to be harmful to a troubled patient ... it is better to reproach a patient that you have saved than to extort money from those who are at death's door.'

The problems with private practice are the same now as they were two millennia ago, but we should know better, and, having experienced seventy-five years of the NHS, be better guarded against them. The degradation of NHS services as they struggle to recover from the onslaught of the pandemic means that many of my patients are now obliged to turn to commercial providers and private clinics because the NHS they've paid into all their lives is no longer able to provide them with a service that's fit for purpose. That must change, and with the right pressure on our political representatives, it can.

The clinical attribute with the greatest currency of all is trust: it's imperative that we continue to feel as if we can trust our doctors and their motivations when they recommend a particular course of treatment. If private providers with profit as their bottom line are allowed to take over, trust evaporates – something I see in my patients who pay for private consultations, listen to a range of their options, then come to me to ask what *I* think they should do, because they know I am paid the same whichever course of action they choose. Removing financial questions from the consulting room and transferring them to a central, government body was one of the most civilised achievements of the twentieth century, perhaps one of the most civilised ideas ever dreamed up by humanity. And if we let our politicians drive profit back into clinical encounters then we haven't moved on since Chaucer, and we're yet to learn from Hippocrates.

6

TOO MUCH MEDICINE: OVERTREATMENT AND OVERDIAGNOSIS

As a newly qualified doctor twenty-five years ago I often did a procedure called a 'pleural tap' – using a needle to drain fluid from the lungs. In the decades since then, research has shown that the more expert you are at pleural taps, the less likely it is that there will be complications such as bleeding, or an injury to the nerve that runs close beneath each rib. In most modern hospitals now you wouldn't get a junior doctor doing a pleural tap – instead a respiratory specialist is called in to do them. But because those specialists are busy on their own wards, the patient can wait for days to have a procedure that can theoretically be completed within minutes. The laudable aim of reducing risk to the patient exposes them to other kinds of less easily definable risks: falls, hospital-acquired infection, deconditioning, social isolation.

In an ideal world we'd all prefer an expert to do every medical procedure, but a lack of tolerance for some kinds of dangers is exposing our patients to others. The hyperspecialisation of medicine is now frequently hindering rather than helping the patient. Several hospital consultants I spoke to this year told me that we need an urgent national conversation about what is 'good enough' medicine, minimising risk to an acceptable level without introducing long hospital stays and long waits for treatment by super-specialists.

If clinicians in the NHS had more time, they would be able to better implement this more realistic approach to medicine, and explore with each patient what the benefits of a particular treatment might be, what their significant risks are, and whether it might actually be better to do nothing. Those conversations take patience, and are inseparable from the proper practice of medicine. When pressed for time it's always easier (and more defensible to a lawyer) to advocate treatment, even when that treatment might not be in your patient's best interests. If we want to roll back overtreatment and all its costs, NHS clinicians need more time.

One of my elderly patients, a delightful housebound lady called Agnes, has very high blood pressure, a condition that puts her at an increased risk of stroke and heart attack. For years I attempted to reduce Agnes's blood pressure and consequently her stroke risk with medications, but after a week or so with each she would call me up and say 'I just can't take those pills, Dr Francis – they make me feel dreadful.' About five years ago I stopped trying. In her mid-nineties now, she's yet to suffer a stroke or a heart attack.

I stopped trying new pills because Agnes didn't want them, and had made an informed choice to take her chances. The effect of the pills is modest, and there's no way of knowing if she personally would be the one whose life would be saved by taking them. But every time I open her medical notes, my computer flashes an alert telling me that I should be doing something about her blood pressure, and prescribe her more pills. Alerts also flash up about her diabetes, her osteoporosis (fragile bones), and her cholesterol levels, which I also have to override. The reason for these alerts is that clinical trials, often funded by drug companies, have shown the benefit of a particular medication in a select population (usually people under seventy-five) who suffer from a single or perhaps two conditions. Those results are then extrapolated to very different populations – older, frailer, more likely to suffer side effects and with multiple complicating conditions – and guidelines are issued urging prescriptions of higher-dose drugs to these broader populations. Only now are we seeing the true costs of this approach.

Agnes doesn't want to ramp up her medications for these age-related conditions. She's unusual: many people, when told they could reduce the risks associated with ageing, readily agree to a prescription – though they might baulk when they realise how tiny the benefit really is. It is common for someone in their eighties now to be taking between ten and twenty pills every day, each one intended to mitigate one risk or another, but bringing their own side effects and interactions.

The reasons for this are complicated. Most GP surgeries are not strictly speaking part of the NHS – they're 'independent contractors' who have only one customer, the local NHS board, who pays them a share of taxpayers' money on behalf of their patients. Broadly speaking they are paid a sum according to how many patients they have and how many different services they offer (as already mentioned, the incentive is to maximise your patient numbers, not to provide continuity of care). The GPs of the practice pay for the upkeep of their premises, heating, lighting and staff salaries, and whatever is left over is what they take as income. Again and again governments have looked at alternative models, but this 'partnership' model has shown itself to be the cheapest to run for the taxpayer. Reliable figures are difficult to come by, but when a practice is taken over by the health board and all its GPs become salaried employees rather than independent contractors, its running costs typically double. That GPs were never taken fully into the NHS but remain outside it as independent contractors has saved the taxpayer billions of pounds over the lifetime of the NHS, but it's a model that's clearly failing, and the way GPs are funded needs fresh thinking as well as more resource if the NHS is to survive. No one would tolerate a system in which surgeons' pay was directly linked to how many patients they could operate on at speed, or whether they used cheaper surgical instruments, or whether they could pay operating room staff less than the going rate, but that's exactly the system we have tolerated in general practice now for seventy-five years.

In 2004 a change in NHS contracts meant that GPs no longer had a legal duty to provide evening and weekend cover for their patients. There were other changes: the money they were given to run their practices became directly linked to how closely the doctors followed prescribing guidelines on blood pressure, cholesterol, diabetes, osteoporosis and dozens of other measurable outcomes – a system known as the Quality and Outcomes Framework ('QOF'). Because GPs are effectively self-employed rather than state employees, close adherence to guidelines became necessary if they were to continue to be able to pay their running costs. Over the fifteen years from 2004 to 2019 the volume of medicines issued by the NHS tripled, as GPs up and down the country began to adhere more closely to these guidelines. It's been estimated that up to 10 per cent of emergency hospital admissions are now related in some way to adverse medication reactions.

To take the example of high blood pressure, Agnes is in a high-risk group, and there's no doubt that reducing her blood pressure would reduce her stroke risk (though it might also make her more light-headed and prone to falls). But the returns on treating modest high blood pressure are poor: with a slight increase in your blood pressure, and no medication, your chance of *not* having a stroke over the course of one study was 97.4 per cent. Taking pills every day only improved those odds to 98.6 per cent. Those figures translate to 17,000 people taking lifelong medication for just fifty of them to see any benefit. That's good if you're one of the fifty (and no one should stop taking their medication without discussion and carefully informing themselves of the risks), but we have no way of telling whether you will be one of the lucky ones to benefit, and 16,950 people will see no benefit and possibly some harm from side effects.

Pharmaceutical companies prefer to cite 'relative' risk over 'absolute' risk reduction because it looks so much more striking to the patient and to the prescriber. If a pill takes the incidence of stroke or heart attack from two in a thousand people to one in a thousand that's a tiny improvement from which 999 people won't benefit, so drug companies often describe it instead as 'halving your risk'

of stroke. The big pharmaceutical companies routinely emphasise figures like these to
manipulate the prescribing of doctors and hike
up the anxieties of patients.

Another example is statins for lowering cholesterol – one study showed that taking statins
might reduce your chance of having a fatal
heart attack by 27 per cent, but when the real
numbers were explored, that's equivalent to
250 people taking 357,000 tablets over five years,
in order to help just *one person*.

Yet another example is diabetes: the number
of people diagnosed with type 2 diabetes has
quadrupled over twenty-five years, partly
because of rising obesity and the widespread
use of processed foods, but also because the
goalposts for diagnosis have moved. Medical
guidelines encourage an aggressive focus on
blood sugar levels in the hope of reducing the
long-term complications of diabetes (dete-
riorating eyesight, kidney problems, blocked
arteries, nerve dysfunction). And for almost
twenty years the QOF system has succeeded in
driving down blood sugar levels nationwide. So

logically, we should expect less of those complications, but there has been 'no increase in life expectancy and quality of life from intensified diabetic therapy', according to John Yudkin of UCL; 'tighter control conferred no benefit in reducing the incidence of coronary mortality, strokes, or total deaths.' It turns out that lowering your glucose levels doesn't improve your survival as much as predicted, but does make you more likely to end up in hospital with a collapse from low blood sugar.

In recent years a series of excellent polemics has been published spelling out just how much doctors and patients have been deceived by Big Pharma at enormous cost to the NHS and to individual patients' lives. James Le Fanu's *Too Many Pills*, Margaret McCartney's *The Patient Paradox* and Ben Goldacre's *Bad Pharma* have all shown how too much medicine is bad medicine. As a medical columnist at the *Telegraph*, Le Fanu has a voluminous mail bag, bringing him hundreds of stories from people who've suffered from this system, though he doesn't take his readers' anecdotal words for it, instead quoting a recent government-sponsored review: 'We have found no definitive evidence that QOF has had any significant effect on emergency admissions or population health or that it is an effective method for reducing inequalities in health and healthcare.'

In Scotland, the QOF was quietly dropped in 2017, and a 'Realistic Medicine' programme was brought in to encourage more personal choice in the clinic room, together with a more balanced interpretation of statistics – each clinician was encouraged to discuss with their patient the Benefits of a treatment, the Risks, the potential Alternatives, and the likely outcomes if they do Nothing ('BRAN'). But thirteen years of telling doctors that if they *don't* prescribe they're both harming their patient *and* they will be financially penalised has established a prescribing culture that will take a long time to roll back. Part of this is because of the UK's rising climate of litigation: what if Agnes has a stroke, and her family decides to sue me for not prescribing her a cocktail of statins and blood pressure drugs? Each time we have a conversation about her medication I have to carefully document that I've discussed the risks of *not* prescribing.

The toxic effects of overdiagnosis and over-treatment have been brought about by the medicalising culture we live in, but also by successive governments who didn't trust doctors' professionalism, and who believed instead that GPs should be paid by results, i.e. by what could be measured on a screen: cholesterol levels, blood pressure readings and number of prescriptions issued. But these are hopeless as markers of good medical care. To undo the damage, doctors and patients are going to have to have faith in one another, and they'll need more time together in the consulting room in order to properly discuss the marginal benefits of medication, and be realistic about the limited power of drugs. Government and healthcare leaders need to reassure both doctors and the patient population that it's often a good idea *not to treat*. The founding ethical principle of medicine is 'First, do no harm'.

★

There have been many criticisms of the Quality Outcomes Framework system that has dominated primary care for almost twenty years: that it deprofessionalises doctors; that it encourages a tick-box approach to medicine; that it leads to diagnosis of conditions that a patient might otherwise never know they had ('overdiagnosis') and the treatment of which might be harmful. But on the whole the scheme was accepted because it was demonstrated that it could improve some aspects of care, and because patients can *choose* whether or not to be involved. Every drug has possible side effects: driving blood sugar too low can make you feel dizzy and weak, and blood-thinning drugs carry a risk of haemorrhage that can be just as devastating as a stroke. Given more time, each GP would be able to explore with each patient how tightly they wish to adhere to 'best practice', discuss which side effects may be acceptable and which wouldn't, and generally tailor their care personally as much as possible.

Drug prescriptions can be stopped, and

treatment plans amended. But allocating new diagnoses to people is something quite different to issuing a prescription. Though a new diagnosis can often be helpful (it can offer access to a community of others similarly affected, and unlock access to support services), it can also stick itself with tenacity to a patient's notes, change the way a patient sees themselves, and the way that others relate to them, for little benefit. This is particularly the case with some mental health diagnoses. One of the oddest episodes of the QOF years was a health secretary intervention in 2017, when Jeremy Hunt rolled out an extra initiative over and above QOF to pay doctors £55 for every diagnosis of dementia that could be inserted into a patient's notes.

As health secretary, Hunt seems to have taken the UK's relatively low diagnosis rate for dementia in comparison with other countries as evidence of poor care rather than poor access to GP and support services. Making a diagnosis of dementia takes time, and scoring tests of memory and cognitive ability can give different results even on consecutive days – no one should receive a diagnosis of something as life-changing as dementia after a single encounter. Instead of examining the reasons why GPs and psychiatrists didn't have enough time with patients experiencing memory loss, or looking into whether poor access to dementia services discourages clinicians from making such a potentially devastating diagnosis, a financial incentive to give diagnoses of 'dementia' was offered as a kind of parallel extension to the idea of payment by results. But paying doctors to make a diagnosis is very different from paying them to maintain high standards.

The dementia initiative of 2017 exposed something crucial at stake about an incentivised way of practising medicine. The extraordinary advances of the last fifty years in public health and specialist care have led to better and better life expectancies. There was a time when if you suffered a heart attack you were given oxygen, morphine and nitroglycerin while doctors waited to see if you lived or died. Now you can expect to be rushed into a cardiac theatre, to have your coronary artery re-expanded with clot-busting drugs and a stent, then to be sent to high-dependency care, perhaps now with an intra-aortic balloon pump or ventricular assist device, possibly after that to receive a bypass graft, before ultimately leaving hospital on five or six new drugs that you'll take for the rest of your life. The massive expansion in the number of people who have survived strokes, heart attacks, cancer or any number of other afflictions, is something we should celebrate. But it also means that GPs spend far more of their time managing the care of patients with chronic disease rather than those needing acute, reactive care. This expansion in the burden of care has taken place without any concomitant transfer in resources.

In 2017 many GPs went on record to say that they would donate any funds they received through dementia diagnosis payments to local services rather than to support their own practices. Perhaps they wished to highlight the paradox that a diagnosis of dementia is of use to you to the extent that it helps you access support, but at the time of its introduction, cuts to local council funding through a programme of government austerity had reduced those services substantially. A diagnosis can also be useful if it gets you a prescription for drugs to help you with your condition, but in the case of dementia there is no such drug – even the latest, very expensive monoclonal antibody treatments offer a very modest benefit (and at time of writing they cost $26,000 dollars per patient per year.) If the dementia is 'moderate', it is claimed that some medications can, in some cases, slow the progress of the disease by about six months – but they don't reverse it, and after six months have 'little or no effect'. The more widely available drugs also have side effects: cramps, exhaustion and insomnia are among those commonly reported.

A month after it was announced, the CEO of NHS England said that the dementia diagnosis payment scheme would be retired. But the damage had been done, and a boundary had been crossed; a cash-for-diagnoses initiative was another example of a medical managerial culture that rewards overdiagnosis and the prescription of drugs over personalised, professional care that takes time.

Recently I sat in on the clinic of a colleague who works as a neurologist specialising in demyelinating conditions such as multiple sclerosis – conditions in which the brain and spinal cord are under attack by the patient's own immune system. The nervous system controls the body and keeps us informed about the world, and so malfunctions of it can manifest in many ways – unsteadiness, dizziness, incontinence, blindness. When I worked in a neurology unit twenty years ago the treatments were relatively crude: we'd use steroids to dampen the reaction of the immune system, and infusions of a naturally occurring protein called interferon which restricts signalling between white blood cells. Since my time on the wards the treatment of the condition has been revolutionised thanks to a slew of new drugs called 'biologics', artificial antibodies designed specifically to slow the pathological process. That day in the MS clinic, patient after patient came through the door with their disease in remission – the consultant had them walking heel-to-toe, hopping on one leg, performing fine dexterous actions with their fingers, demonstrating just how well these drugs had kept their disease in abeyance.

'These drugs really are so much better for patients,' she told me, 'but I *do* worry about how expensive they are.' Regular infusions of a drug called ocrelizumab, one of the most widely prescribed, costs the NHS (and so the taxpayer) around £20,000 a year per patient. Biologic therapies are transforming the treatment of many other conditions: inflammatory bowel disease, rheumatoid arthritis, migraine and osteoporosis, to name just a few. Adalimumab, which can be used for rheumatoid arthritis but also for ulcerative colitis and psoriasis, was at one point the most expensive drug for the NHS, costing the taxpayer £400 million a year (or around £8,600 per patient in receipt of it). When adalimumab came off patent in 2018 that bill dropped by almost 40 per cent. But it remained a very expensive drug. As more and more conditions become amenable to treatment by biologic therapies, the NHS drug bill is going to soar.

I'm not aware that any political party is proposing amendment to the rules on how many years companies can hold the patent over new drugs, and so the prices of the latest life-enhancing medications will continue to be set by pharmaceutical companies rather than the market for many decades to come. The money for these drugs will need to be found somewhere if the principles of the NHS are to remain intact, and if people in the UK are to have access to the best of modern healthcare. Many clinicians fear that we're already into a two-tier medical culture – something that happened in dentistry many years ago – whereby one level of treatment can be accessed by those who can pay, while a basic, catch-all level using poorer drugs and materials will become the norm for patients within the NHS. But getting a cheaper metal filling in your tooth has very different consequences to having substandard treatment for your multiple sclerosis.

Most of my own patients, if they are going to benefit personally from the prescription of a drug, are convinced that it should be provided by the NHS no matter its cost. But when those costs are paid out to benefit others, some begin to question their value, and adherence to the NHS's principles begin to weaken. 'It's because we're keeping the old folk alive too long', one patient told me, when I apologised over how long she'd have to wait to be seen. 'It's because of all those managers', said another, unswayed by my insistence that the NHS is among the most efficient healthcare systems in the world, its management bill very low in comparison with that of other countries, never mind its huge efficiency over other industries and services.

To get around this question of which drugs are simply too expensive for the NHS to afford, the UK government of 1997 set up a body, the National Institute of Clinical Excellence (NICE), whose specialists worked to a benchmark of agreeing to any drug that for £20,000–£30,000 would offer, on average, a year of life saved that could be lived at good quality. These 'QALYs' (Quality Adjusted Life Years) are by necessity controversial – open to interpretation and manipulation by pharmaceutical companies keen for their medicines to be available on the NHS, and willing to set prices at a level where they'll be highly profitable but still within the threshold of NICE. For all its flaws the principle seems an effective compromise, balancing the needs of patients with the need to balance the books.

In February 2023, a gene therapy for metachromatic leukodystrophy (MLD), a rare disorder of children's metabolism affecting around 1 in 100,000 live births, was approved for use in the NHS. Libmeldy treatment involves extracting bone marrow stem cells from the affected child, using chemotherapy to wipe out the function of their remaining bone marrow, altering the genetic makeup of the extracted stem cells using viral DNA technology, and reinfusing those stem cells back into the patient. When effective it offers a permanent cure, and the list price of £2.8 million set a record for a drug treatment prescribed on the NHS.

In this case the costs were approved for NHS use because of the permanence of the potential cure, and because those costs could be offset against the substantial costs of treating an affected child with such a debilitating and ultimately fatal condition. For the child and her family the treatment was indisputably worthwhile, and many taxpayers will applaud it. Yet it's clear that the NHS doesn't have nearly enough resource to do all that is currently being asked of it. Patients left waiting for years with milder but life-limiting or disabling conditions amenable to cheaper treatments will argue that the money could have been better spent on staff or on hospital capacity.

The NHS drugs budget makes up only a tiny proportion of the tax spend on the NHS, and the body NHS Improvement didn't even mention it in its recent list of eleven urgent priorities for NHS reform.* But those costs

---

* Though a 'budget impact test' has recently been

are significant – the taxpayer spends £309 per patient per year on drugs, almost double the entire primary care budget of just £181 per year per patient (having access to a GP costs about the same per person as having a TV licence).

The questions of which expensive and innovative drugs and treatments should be provided by the NHS isn't up to doctors, but to voters – how generous a national drug bill are they willing to support? As scientists learn more about illness and how to tackle it, and increasingly costly treatments become available, we need a public conversation about which interventions, as a society, we're prepared to fund. Right now we're not even having a conversation about what we can *stop doing*, never mind which drugs we can and cannot afford. We need a national debate, perhaps through a series of citizens' assemblies, on what the taxpayer is prepared to pay for. If no more money is forthcoming, a decision needs to be made.

---

introduced into the assessment of any drug that might cost the NHS more than £20 million.

Do we want more access to innovative drugs, or do we want more time with our doctors? The current settlement means it's not possible to have both.

In conversations with specialist consultants I often hear that their attempts to introduce more realistic conversations with their patients about the marginal benefit of very expensive drugs are stymied by patient expectations. 'Society has become more obsessed with tests and new drugs', one told me. 'They have a shaky grasp of how perilously close to failure the whole system is; explaining the true pros and cons of any new treatment takes time, and it's always easier to over-investigate and overtreat because it meets those inflated expectations, and it's quicker to arrange than taking the time to patiently go through the small benefits and potential risks of a new treatment. But it's not necessarily best for the patient.' Another put it more simply: 'politicians need to be a lot more honest with the voters that there are things that we can and cannot afford.'

7

FRAILTY AND SOCIAL CARE: A MAGNIFICENT SUCCESS STORY

Lifespans around the world more than doubled through the twentieth century – from an average of just thirty-two years in 1900, to sixty-six in 2000. At the founding of the NHS in 1948 men in the UK lived to just sixty-six on average, and women to seventy-one. In just a few decades, humanity's life expectancy improved by more than it had over the preceding 10,000 years. Before the Covid dip of 2020 that figure had reached seventy-two worldwide, and, in Europe, seventy-nine. This is a magnificent success story. So why is it that seniority, age and frailty are seen as a problem for society, rather than a cause for celebration? The answer must be the economy: in terms of costs to the NHS the average sixty-five-year-old has double the healthcare costs of a thirty-year-old, and an eighty-five-year-old costs five times as much. It's between the ages of thirty and sixty-four that people are more likely to have private health insurance – the very years in which healthcare tends to be least needed.

Hospital clinicians make a distinction between the 'front door' of the hospital – A&E, Acute Receiving Units, GP admission requests, which as we've already seen are becoming over-whelmed by demand – and the 'back door' of the hospital, which patients pass through on their way home. To keep movement flowing through the front *and* back door a number of moving parts have to work together: discharge medications need to be made up; prescription alterations communicated to the GP; frail, unsteady people need to be assessed to ensure they can manage safely around their own home; arrangements for social care need to be put in place for those who can't wash themselves, prepare food or get to the toilet; and outpatient appointments need to be made for specialist follow-up. The drift towards a more atomised society, where fewer people have family support close by, has made the question of social care progressively more pressing, and many of my middle-aged patients are now being forced to become carers for their elderly parents in a way that they hadn't expected. Most of the discharge planning work to get people from hospital to home isn't done by nurses or doctors, but by physiotherapists, occupational therapists, pharmacists and social workers. Some are employed by the NHS, and some are employed by the local council. Despite valiant efforts at creating joint boards in much of the country, the lack of joined-up thinking (and budgets) between a national body like the NHS and local council bodies is one of many reasons that social care in the UK is failing.

Recently a friend of mine who works as a general physician told me that in her large general hospital there's now just one physiotherapist to cover three medical wards – one person to cover a *hundred patients*. One day extra in hospital costs the NHS about £350 per patient, while a physiotherapist's salary is around £30,000 a year – perhaps NHS budget holders have done the mathematics and have concluded that it's cheaper to keep people in hospital than it is to provide enough physiotherapists to help get them home?

My first home visit of the day was a ninety-seven-year-old woman who just 'wasn't right'. Her daughter phoned about ten, while I was still doing the morning clinic. Between patients I'd noticed her name pop up on the screen. 'What do you mean, "not right",' I asked Pearl, the receptionist, on my way to call someone from the waiting room. 'Just that,' she shrugged, '"not right"'.

I visit Betty Cruikshank every month or so. She lives with her disabled daughter Norma in a two-up two-down, spending most of her day on a bed in the back room. There are crash mats around the bed wired to alarms, because

Betty is adept at getting over the high rails fitted to her bedframe. Even so, a while ago she fell out of bed and lay for an hour before she was found, with her ankle tangled in the rails. She has dementia, has suffered a couple of strokes, but she manages to eat the food that the council's carers or Norma put down before her, and she cooperates, for the most part, with attempts to keep her clean.

It was true – she wasn't right. 'Hello, Mrs Cruikshank,' I bellowed in her ear, and she took a long time about replying. When she did her words were more slurred than usual, and she seemed to look over my shoulder rather than at me. She wouldn't lift her arm or show me her tongue when I asked her to, and I heard an ominous rattling sound when I put my stethoscope to her chest. She was breathing faster than usual.

'She's spluttering when she drinks,' volunteered her daughter, who used to work as a carer. 'Could she have had another stroke?'

'She might have', I said, 'or she might just be more confused from a chest infection.'

Betty has had a 'Do Not Attempt Resuscitation' form in place for years, though she's gone in and out of hospital from time to time for chest infections, and once for kidney failure consequent to dehydration. 'We could admit her for a scan,' I added, 'to see if she's had a stroke, but I don't think that's in her best interests.' I paused to gauge her daughter's expression, to see whether she might be about to accuse me of ageism. 'But to be honest, I think she'd be happier if we keep her here, and try treating the infection.' Norma nodded, with obvious relief. 'I don't think she'd want to go to hospital,' she said. If her daughter hadn't lived with her, Betty would have had to have been admitted – carers from the council come in for just a few minutes at a time, at most four times a day.

I had just strapped my briefcase to the rack of my bicycle when the phone in my pocket went. It was Pearl: 'Are you still out?' she asked. 'Mary Robertson's just phoned, she says she can't breathe.' I put the waiting room anger out of my mind – another visit now meant I'd be at least half an hour late starting afternoon clinic – and summoned what I could remember of Mary Robertson. I knew her less well: a fit ninety-two-year-old widow who lived alone in a sheltered housing complex, still managing her own shopping and with a carer who came in once a day to help and whom she paid for out of her own funds. I remembered bladder problems, hip pain, but couldn't summon much else.

Her voice sounded breathless and panicked on the entry phone; she pushed a button and let me into the complex. Inside: pastel walls hung with innocuous prints, hard-wearing carpets and stairs edged with metal footplates. Her door was open and I pushed my way into a meticulously clean apartment, red alarm cords hanging from the ceilings, each wired to a central office with a telephonist on duty. Mary wore an alarm button on a pendant around her neck; she sat perched on the edge of her settee, breathing hard, with dread in her eyes.

She'd been getting more and more breathless for the last two days. No, she hadn't had any chest pain, no her ankles hadn't been swelling. She had low oxygen saturations of 92 per cent, her breathing rate was too fast, and her pulse rate was well over a hundred. On the left side of her chest I heard air moving normally, but the right side was practically silent. When I tapped her chest it sounded hollow on the left, but on the right it was like tapping a stone.

'I think you've got water on one lung,' I said, taking a seat beside her on the sofa. She was using her hands to push against her thighs, the better to lift her shoulders into each breath. 'We can drain it off,' I said, 'but you'd need to go to the hospital for that.'

'If you say so, son,' Mary replied. I didn't know the reason for the fluid build-up – it could be a sign of tumour in the lung, could be heart failure, could be any number of other disturbances of her ninety-two-year-old equilibrium. But without active treatment she would soon be dead.

Afternoon clinic was unremarkable: twelve patients allotted just ten minutes each; a relatively rewarding assortment of fevers, injuries, anxieties, aches and despondencies. I was half an hour late in starting and I didn't make up the time. When I'd written up the last consultation, and was just about to read the hospital correspondence, there was a knock at the door – Pearl again. 'I'm really sorry, Gavin, there's another visit request. Ellen MacIvor's carer has phoned, says she's confused.'

Ellen MacIvor was a ninety-five-year-old woman who, amazingly enough, still lived alone on the second floor of an old tenement. She'd never married, but had a niece who dropped by three times a week. Council carers visited three times a day to help her with meals, but Ellen was able to wash and dress herself and even prepare some food. When I'd first met her, seven years earlier, she managed the stairs with ease, but I suspected that for the last year or so she'd hardly been out.

The keys to her building were held in a safe box screwed to the tenement stairwell entrance; I punched in the code and two keys dropped out. I let myself in, negotiated the baby buggies and bicycles padlocked to the landings, and used the second key to gain entry to the flat. 'Miss MacIvor,' I shouted from the door, but there was no answer. Worn carpets, spilled food on the skirting boards. I went through to the living room: she was sleeping on an easy chair in front of an electric fire. A sandwich left by the lunchtime carers was untouched, and a note from them said they'd tried to get her up to the toilet, but she couldn't walk. I worked once with a hospital physician who called this 'acopia', because the main symptom is 'inability to cope'. I worked with another who called it 'de-pedism', because the patient has 'gone off their feet'.

'Miss MacIvor!', I shouted a bit more loudly. Her eyes opened slowly; like Betty, who I'd seen at lunchtime, she looked absently over my shoulder instead of at me. Also like Betty, her chest sounded terrible – full of phlegm and whistling with wheeze. She was able to give me her name and date of birth, but got her age, address and the year wrong when I questioned her. She too had a chest infection, and if she could be supported at home with antibiotics as Betty had, she had a good chance of being able to avoid hospital admission. But there was no hoisting equipment in the flat to move her, no diagnostic equipment beyond my stetho- scope, thermometer and oxygen saturation probe, and it was by now 7 p.m. There was no mechanism for me to arrange carers to come in overnight.

On the windowsill I found a care plan with a phone number for her niece. 'She needs some antibiotics and some tests,' I said down the phone. A nervous, pained voice answered: 'In the hospital?'

'Not necessarily,' I replied, 'are you nearby?'

'No – not back for another couple of days,' she said.

'I could try to get the carers doubled up,' I said, though none of that could happen until the following morning. 'And if we get four visits a day instead of three, we might be able to keep her here while I treat her chest infection.'

'I'd worry about that, doctor,' she replied. 'She'll try to get up, and she'll fall. I don't think we can take the risk.'

I phoned the hospital, arranged the ambulance, wrote up the referral letter and left it propped at the door entrance, on top of a little pile of papers and blister packs, where the ambulance crew would see it as soon as they came in. 'You're going to the hospital,' I said to Miss MacIvor. Her eyes opened: 'Oh no, oh no', she murmured, before nodding back to sleep.

My first patient of the day, Betty, was lucky – she had a daughter who could take the decision with me not to prolong her life by all means possible, and a social care package that could be tweaked to keep her at home. The second patient, Mary, was the kind of nonagenarian hospital managers like: fit and independent, with one presenting complaint that they could diagnose, treat and discharge – indeed, she went home with further tests arranged as an outpatient. But it's patients like Ellen, my third patient of the day, that the NHS doesn't know how to deal with. She ended up in hospital for weeks, getting more and more institutionalised, less and less able to manage on her own – 'blocking a bed'. But to unblock her bed there would have to be massive investment in social care, and the creation of a truly twenty-four-hour care service that's able to come to her home day or night, at short notice, get her washed and into bed, arrange streamlined transport for any X-rays or scans that she needs, and double her provision of carers for as long as she requires them. Another alternative is that we reopen a series of intermediate care hospitals and cottage hospitals to which GPs can admit patients to keep them away from A&E. But we're a long way from that kind of service: on a recent lunchtime home visit I phoned the urgent care service for a similar case, hoping to avoid a patient's admission, and was told 'it's after 1 p.m. You should have called before noon.'

To take pressure off the hospitals we need dramatic investment in a new kind of primary care in the community, employing enough carers that they can be rapidly deployed to help keep elderly people out of hospital, as well as far more district nurses, who already do much to prevent emergency admissions but are woefully undervalued. Their numbers are falling through early retirements, short-sighted withdrawal of training and bursaries, and because a tipping point has been reached: increasingly impossible rotas are encouraging more and more of them to quit.

When the voters are told that there's not enough money for a functioning NHS and social care system, my reply is 'that's actually not true'. France, Germany, Sweden and Denmark all spend more than the UK on healthcare, and there is nothing constitutionally different about our people or economy that we can't spend on health and well-being to the same level as our neighbours. Instead, there has been a political decision not to adequately fund care here. A little extra funding in social care could be transformative for the failing NHS.

8

IDENTIFYING PROBLEMS, EXPLORING SOLUTIONS

Individual health is inextricable from planetary health, and globally, healthcare causes around 4 per cent of carbon emissions. Good healthcare is also lower-carbon healthcare: energy-efficient buildings have cheaper running costs, saving more public money for medical care. Good management of chronic conditions leads to fewer hospital admissions and fewer drug prescriptions – all of which has a carbon cost as well as a personal and financial cost. As the NHS recovers from thirteen years of underfunding, that rebuilding effort should be carried out with more care of the environment than has been customary so far, and with greater honesty than simply headline-grabbing initiatives such as the Nightingale Hospitals (which could never have had enough staff to be fit for purpose), or pledges of building infrastructure that politicians have no intention of fulfilling (such as a recent government promise to build forty new hospitals).

Private finance initiative (PFI) projects of the 1990s resulted in hospital services, such as canteens and car parks, that local management teams have no control over, and a bill to the taxpayer that the National Audit Office has estimated at 70 per cent higher than it would have been had the government simply borrowed to build projects itself. That is money that could have been spent on patient care. A health service finance executive told me recently that her hospital car park had changed hands four times since the PFI contract was signed, and was now owned by an equities firm based in Switzerland.

A King's Fund report in August 2022 stated that 'from 2014/15 to 2019/20, funds from capital budgets were transferred to support day-to-day spending and relieve the growing pressures in the NHS'. Funds that were meant to maintain the NHS's bricks and mortar were diverted away from their intended purpose, leaving a £9 billion backlog in maintenance bills. In this book I've tried to outline a few ways in which the NHS is ailing, and rebuilding its infrastructure with the environment in mind must be one of its highest priorities. At the outset of the NHS Bevan wrote to the medical profession: 'My job is to give you all the facilities, resources and help I can, and then to leave you alone as professional men and women to use your skill and judgement without hindrance.' Doctors and nurses are now unable to use skill or judgement without hindrance. We are being hindered.

For the NHS to flourish, we need better mechanisms of establishing what works well and what doesn't – without having to contract in expensive management consultants and think tanks with obscure funding arrangements. New ideas that have helped one corner of the service could be rolled out to other areas with far more agility than they are currently. The kind of transformation we need is possible if we develop mechanisms that enable us to learn from our successes as well as our mistakes.

Jeremy Hunt is the longest-serving health secretary the UK has ever seen. He wrote in a recent memoir that lives in the NHS are being shortened avoidably because of its blame culture, short staffing and underfunding. His book is illustrated with examples that offer a measure of calculated candour about his own party's culpability in defunding the service, about neglectful workforce planning, and the stripping of resources from social care. One in ten NHS patients is at risk of some sort of avoidable harm as a result of NHS treatment. While these figures may be unacceptable they are comparable to those of other healthcare systems and are not unique to the NHS – a consequence of an overstrained service as well as the complexity of modern healthcare, in which patients live for decades with conditions that once killed within weeks. Hunt later became Chancellor of the Exchequer and so might be expected to have promptly put in place the funding for one of his principal prescriptions for the NHS: more staff, and thus more continuity of care. He also counselled greater transparency and accountability at all levels as a way of driving improvements in the quality of care. They are good ambitions, and as I read his memoir I found myself nodding, looking forward to his insistence on the same values among fellow MPs.

The unintended consequences of a blame culture, finding fault with individual nurses and doctors for systemic or structural issues, are what prompted one of the most egregious episodes in NHS history in the last twenty years – the Mid-Staffordshire scandal, in which a culture of neglect and denial flourished under a management obsessed with New Labour targets to the detriment of patient care. Staff were ordered not to speak out about failures of care, and nurses were threatened with the sack if A&E waiting times breached four hours, and then, when records were found to have been amended to keep to target, were sacked anyway.* The inquiry turned up several examples of medical and nursing negligence, yet most of those called to give evidence cited cuts from management and understaffing as the cause of those failures. The Mid-Staffs scandal (as it came to be known) sounded a warning; we know that the Trust's negligence went on for so long because there were inadequate avenues for clinicians to blow the whistle on dangerous care. A national service was set up for staff to raise concerns: each health board area now has a dedicated team whose job it is to invite and investigate staff concerns over potentially dangerous inadequacies in standards of care. Health boards are obliged to take these staff concerns into account, and to explore solutions.

Last winter, a friend of mine who works as

---

* See Isabel Hardman's *Fighting for Life* and Roger Taylor's *God Bless the NHS* for thorough descriptions of the Mid-Staffs scandal.

an acute hospital physician told me that her
department often felt like a war zone in which
she was simply triaging as quickly as possible
without time to think in a deep or systematic way about her patients' problems. There
simply wasn't enough space on the ward for
all the patients that needed hospital treatment,
and standards were dropping as a result. At the
same time another friend, who is a journalist,
asked me how things really were in the hospitals at the front line of the winter crisis. It
made sense to me that the two of them speak
to one another, and with the Mid-Staffs scandal
in mind I suggested an introduction – purely
so that news about the real difficulties and
dangers of our hospitals could get out. 'Can't
do it,' my friend said, 'any contact from a journalist has to go through the health board's press
team.' Contractually, most hospital doctors
are not allowed to speak to the press. If they
have concerns about standards they are told to
either speak to the local whistleblowing team,
or if they are unsatisfied with the response
they get (and in my own health board area,

letters of concern submitted anonymously are not investigated), they should contact the national whistleblowing service. Which means that more than a decade after the Mid-Staffs scandal, many hospital staff are still contractually forbidden from speaking to journalists or those outside health governance when they have concerns over poor quality care.

The airline trade, the building trade, the nuclear industry – all of these have developed effective mechanisms of reporting on unsafe practices and addressing dangerous performance, because the consequences of failure are so stark. But NHS failures are no less dangerous, and the consequences of those failures no less stark. The 'Winter pressures' letter that the Chief Medical Officers of the UK sent to all the doctors in the country in late 2022 stated that 'It is the responsibility of all providers commissioned by the NHS and healthcare leaders to ensure that all clinicians working in their organisations are well supported in their work, and that channels for raising and acting on concerns remain open and accessible to all staff.' But that same letter stated 'It is, and is going to remain, hard going'. It's not at all clear which dangerous inadequacies of care should be reported, and which should be accepted as 'hard going'. When I have tried to point out episodes of seriously inadequate care in my own area, I've been told by senior clinicians that they're very sorry, but that there aren't the resources to do things any better, and so my concerns will have to remain unaddressed. Given that the Chief Medical Officers have told the workforce that they're aware the service can't cope, and that the Chief Executive Officer of NHS England has already told the government the NHS is underfunded and can't meet demand, I should simply accept them as 'hard going'.

Transparency should be a pillar of effective democracy, and when an experienced former health secretary and skilled politician like Jeremy Hunt insists that the NHS needs more transparency, I applaud his intention. This book is in part an attempt to meet that expectation, to point out some of the problems I see in day-to-day practice, and to make modest suggestions as to how they might be addressed in order to save the NHS.

In Scotland the health secretary's official title is 'Cabinet Secretary for NHS Recovery, Health and Social Care', acknowledging that the NHS is in dire straits and in need of convalescence. At the time of writing the secretary is Michael Matheson, a former occupational therapist with first-hand experience of many of the problems outlined in this book, particularly the lack of joined-up thinking between hospital and social care. In May 2023 I sat on a panel event in Ullapool with one of his predecessors, Jeane Freeman (health minister from 2018 to 2021), and Linda Bauld, Professor of Public Health at Edinburgh University. As panellists, we were asked, respectively, to share first-hand clinical experiences, offer political perspectives, and make international comparisons with regard to Scotland's response to Covid. In the course of the conversation I said that the NHS was failing so severely that the four Chief Medical

Officers of the UK now expected clinical standards to worsen over winter, and I didn't know
why that change hadn't been front-page news.
The journalist Ruth Wishart, who was chairing
our conversation, laughed and replied that she
wondered how far we would get into the discussion before journalists would get the blame
for the problems of the NHS. I laughed too –
after all journalists are clearly not to blame for
the failures of the NHS – but there's no doubt
that journalism is vital to the way a democracy
works, letting the electorate understand what
is going on at government level, and the impact
government choices have on public services.

The NHS benefits from transparency, but
transparency also needs a media culture that's
able to dispassionately assess the evidence,
something often lacking in news reporting that
covers health matters. An example of regretta-
ble media standards during the Covid pandemic
was the way in which staff in many care homes
where there was an outbreak of Covid were
harassed by press photographers, with the care
home rapidly becoming front-page news. This

was at a time when Covid testing was still very inaccurate, and only around 60 per cent sensitive: in other words, if a hundred people with Covid had been discharged to care homes from hospital, careful testing would only have identified infection in sixty of them. Forty would still have been discharged into care homes, and able to spread the virus.

We have a system with zero slack, and so there was never anywhere else for these patients with Covid to go but into care homes. The hospitals didn't have any spare capacity, there was insufficient staff even for the Nightingale Hospitals, and by definition these were people who weren't able to live independently. The reaction of most care homes was to further isolate some of the most isolated people in our communities. One elderly couple in a care home I look after, *who were married*, were confined to separate rooms, not allowed to see one another for months, because care managers were so terrified of becoming front-page news that they banned *any* interaction between residents.

Unbiased information about the problems of the NHS is available for those who would like to find it, and recently a journalist at the *Financial Times*, John Burn-Murdoch, investigated and then reported on how many of the problems of the NHS are due to systematic underfunding and an economy that is performing worse than that of our European neighbours. 'If you're lucky, you can get away with cutting investment for a few years,' Burn-Murdoch wrote. 'Everything gets a bit more fragile, but as long as there are no nasty external shocks, you might be able to avoid disaster. The effects of slashing public services are a little harder to hide, but you might get away with gradual deterioration.' He goes on:

> The problem is, when you're hit by a pandemic, an energy crisis and an act of gross economic self-sabotage in short order, your now brittle and exhausted public services will buckle where a healthy system would have taken the strain. Twelve years on from the start of austerity, the data paint a

damning picture, from stagnant wages and frozen productivity to rising chronic illness and a health service on its knees.

Burn-Murdoch's article was accompanied by graphs with the following headings, which speak for themselves: 'The Tories' austerity programme made deep and lasting cuts to public spending, especially investment, eroding Britain's state capacity'; 'UK real wages are lower today than 18 years ago, and have fared much worse than any peer nation'; 'The impacts have been stark, from ballooning waiting lists and worsening A&E performance, to a rise in avoidable deaths and stalling life expectancy.' If the striking graphs from this article were shown on television, or more widely in the press, including the tabloid media, it's my impression that our politicians would feel a greater pressure to fund the NHS to the standards that the voters expect.

The UK has a relatively low rate of litigation against doctors in comparison with some countries; even so, payouts to those who sue the NHS represent a substantial cost to the service. The budget for the NHS in England this year is £153 billion, and negligence claims are now more than £2 billion a year, much of this going to the lawyers who pursue those claims in court (when searching for these figures online, I was beset by advertisements offering no-win no-fee services to help me sue the NHS). Since early 2022 the government has been attempting to introduce a cap on legal costs to control this, and in a formal report commented: 'The overall cost of clinical negligence in England rose from £582 million in 2006–7 to £2.2 billion in 2020–21, representing a significant burden on the NHS. For all claims, legal costs have increased more than fourfold to £433 million since 2006–7.'

It has been calculated that the typical GP makes about ten thousand clinical judgements over the course of a year. GP and writer Phil Whitaker points out that even a very good doctor who makes the right call 99 per cent of the time is still going to get something wrong about a hundred times a year. If just 1 per cent of those mistakes turn out to be dangerous ones, even a very good GP will make a significant, potentially fatal mistake, *every year* that they are in practice – and that is for the very best and most careful doctors, practising in a system that is well resourced. Medicine in its best manifestations should be able to support clinicians to be the best that they can be, and help them find ways of learning from their mistakes rather than driving those doctors out of the profession. I'd like to see a National Health Service that supports all clinicians, doctors, nurses and allied health professionals to act in the best interests of their patients, to learn from their mistakes, but to be protected from the kind of career-wrecking and budget-wrecking medical negligence industry that flourishes in some parts of the world. New Zealand has an entirely different system: called 'no-fault compensation' it provides support and reparations to people who have suffered side effects or injury as a result of medical treatment, and does so without deepening a culture of blame.

It is far easier for patients to navigate, and fairer for everyone involved. In the UK we have a service now that is so stressed that mistakes have become inevitable, and a system like that of New Zealand would offer the best of both worlds as we rebuild the NHS: a service that can fully support its clinicians to learn from mistakes, yet compensate any patients that have come to harm.

One of the most radical ways that some pressure could be taken off front-line NHS services, and free up some breathing space, is for health promotion and public health initiatives to be taken out of the clinic room and put back into the hands of government. Regular exercise, a good diet, smoking cessation, alcohol awareness, screening programmes – all of these things are important for the health of the nation, but my days as a GP are now so pressured that it's impossible for me to take all of these on as my role and still be a good doctor. To get better value for money from the salaries of NHS clinicians, health managers should now think carefully about which parts of the service need doctors and which parts can be done by other professionals.

The responsibility to deliver the Covid vaccination programme is a good example. It was clearly going to be impossible for GP surgeries to take on the vaccination of the entire population while continuing to see patients, and so the usual way of funding a new community service – offer GPs some money and ask them to do it on top of the rest of their work – was dismissed out of hand, and an alternative way of providing that service was found. One of the most transformative initiatives of recent years in terms of improving my workload and offering patients a better service was the introduction to many GP surgeries of 'community link workers', highly skilled people who are trained not in medicine or in nursing but in helping patients access the right kinds of support in terms of housing, benefits and mental health. Because community link workers aren't also trying to manage urgent presentations of illness, and stay abreast of the latest medical guidelines and research, they are more able to keep up with the latest services available locally.

As we have seen, Bevan regarded the family doctor as possibly the most important person in the National Health Service. 'He comes into the most immediate and continuous touch with the members of the community. He is also the gateway to all the other branches of the Service. If more is required than he can provide, it is he who puts the patient in touch with the specialist services. He is also the most highly individualistic member of the medical world.' GPs provide an extraordinarily good service in terms of value for money, but demand has overwhelmed the number of appointments available and there are not enough GPs coming through to do what's asked of them. In a ten-minute appointment I'm routinely asked to deal with three or four different problems (my record so far is nine). For the NHS to be saved, general practice needs to survive. Large parts of what we ask GPs to do can be done by other members of the wider healthcare team. Though my love for the job is in large part a love for the breadth and richness and diversity of my working day, it's urgent that we ask of each encounter: which of these tasks requires someone with a medical degree and ten years of training, and which tasks can be done by somebody else?

9

SAVE OUR SERVICE

No society can legitimately call itself
civilized if a sick person is denied
medical aid because of lack of means.

Aneurin Bevan, *In Place of Fear*

More than seventy-five years ago Aneurin Bevan
wrote an open letter to the medical profession
inaugurating the new National Health Service.
'On 5 July we start, together,' he wrote. 'There
have been understandable anxieties, inevitable
in so great and novel an undertaking. Nor will
there be overnight any miraculous removal
of our more serious shortages of nurses and
others and of modern replanned buildings and
equipment. But the sooner we start, the sooner

we can try together to see to these things and to secure the improvements we all want.' The spirit of the letter was one of collaboration, though he was aware that there would be problems ahead. 'Doubtless other defects can be found and further improvements made', he wrote, four years after the service opened. 'What emerges, however, in the final count, is the massive contribution the British Health Service makes to the equipment of a civilized society. It has now become a part of the texture of our national life.'

So how do we save our service? As one consultant physician put it to me: 'It's surely not beyond our wit to come up with a better way.' Let us honour the principles that established the NHS, a healthcare service that's free for all, funded by the people, for the people. The alternative is to return to the days of keeping a jar of money aside for doctors' bills, and living in fear of illness. Find ways of supporting community care, which sees 90 per cent of the patients with less than 10 per cent of the funding. People who have known their GP for years, and can get a non-urgent appointment to see them, have 30 per cent lower admission rates to hospital than those who don't know their GP – and they live longer too. Let's ask our elected representatives to benchmark the NHS against comparable European countries and insist that they commit to funding our service adequately, so that it can keep up. The voters are more unhappy with the NHS than they've been for thirty years, so let's listen to them, and change it for the better. To say that a functioning NHS is unaffordable is to admit to a startling lack of faith in civilised society.

Many front-line clinicians said of the winter of 2022–23 that it was the worst they can remember, and we need to urgently expand hospital wards as well as community care capacity in order to cope with the patient numbers that need help each winter. A system that's fit only for summer is a system that's not fit at all. Healthcare is people work and it needs investment in people – not only by restoring their wages but also by training them, celebrating them, and trusting in their professionalism.

Morale among clinical staff is shockingly low, and there are hundreds of unexplored ways that the mood and working conditions in our hospitals and our clinics could be improved. The caring professions in Britain right now could do with a bit of care – and some hope. It's not so long ago that we were clapping them from the doorsteps; let's now show them some of that support.

The service can't do all of what is being asked of it right now, so let's start an urgent national conversation, perhaps through citizens' assemblies, about what its priorities should be. What can the depleted workforce *stop doing* to free up capacity and time? How much health promotion can be transferred out of the clinic room and onto TV, radio, billboards? And how much of a drugs budget are the voters willing to support – the current settlement means it's not possible to have every treatment that every patient might want. Cherish generalism, and ask of the specialists: what standards are 'good enough' to get the best level of care to the greatest number of people? Because by focusing on stratospheric standards in some areas we have let others fall to appallingly low levels. Don't be fooled by the brochures and promises of private healthcare companies, whose profits are bolstered when the NHS is struggling, even though the service regularly helps them to manage their own failures. Most private doctors in the UK are also NHS doctors, and no one wants decisions about their clinical care made by shareholders. Clinicians need more time with their patients to have conversations about what the marginal benefits of many treatments really are, and whether giving a formal diagnosis is always appropriate. If we could have honest discussions about the benefits, risks and alternatives to many treatments, there's a good chance we'd do fewer of them.

Until the downturn in life expectancy caused by Covid and by policies of austerity, people were living longer than they've ever lived in the history of humanity. In a caring, civilised society, having an ageing population needn't be a burden, but could instead be something worth celebrating. Let's build a network of home care teams and intermediate care hospitals that can keep the frail and the elderly away from trolleys on corridors and queues in A&E, finding ways of looking after them closer to home with dignity and compassion.

Planetary health is inextricable from individual health: as the NHS recovers it has to find ways to build back better, with the environmental impact of its buildings and its drugs in mind. Less waste and more efficient buildings save money that can be used for patient care. Mistakes are inevitable in any system of healthcare, and a less litigious way of assessing compensation would help patients who have been harmed as well as helping clinicians learn from mistakes – as well as the NHS budget. Just as journalists should be able to find out the truth of what's happening in the health service, the health service should be able to depend on reliable and unbiased reporting of its successes as well as its failures. The stakes around the way we talk about the NHS couldn't be higher – our democracy as well as the health of almost 70 million people depend on it.

★

At a teaching session recently at my local medical school a disconsolate and anxious group of students asked me about falling standards in the NHS, dismal morale among clinicians, and whether there could be any hope for their own careers. 'We look at the junior doctors,' one said, 'and wonder what it is that we've signed up for.' I told them that thirty years ago when I started out in medicine the feeling in the NHS was the same: a burned-out, exhausted workforce was fed up of working in a failing, underfunded service. Patient dissatisfaction was at an unprecedented high when, towards the end of my university training, there was a change of government. The voters demonstrated that they wanted their politicians to put the NHS back to the top of the priority list, and taxpayers' money flooded in. Morale among doctors, nurses and allied professionals began quickly to rise, and patient satisfaction too; within a few years of the change studies were being published that put the NHS among the most effective and efficient healthcare services in the developed world. 'The disenchantment in the NHS now won't last forever,' I said to those students. 'The fortunes of the NHS will improve again, they have to.' I told them that despite all of the challenges of the service as it is today, caring for others remains the most rewarding of jobs; to work in medicine or nursing is to engage your intellect, your curiosity, your humanity, your compassion, and there's no other job I'd want to do.

The principles on which the NHS was founded are still widely revered – good-quality healthcare for all, provided by everybody, *for* everybody. Whether those principles can continue to stand up against the costs of a twenty-first-century world of gene therapy, robotic surgery, innovative biologic treatments and stem cell transplants, and a population that's living longer (and with more frailty) than it has ever done, remains to be seen – but I'm optimistic that it can. The alternative is to admit to a lack of imagination and compassion. A health service free for all at the point of use, based on need rather than on demand, is an expression of what's best in our society, and we'll get the NHS we're prepared to insist on. I hope you'll agree that it's worth saving.

BRITISH MEDICAL JOURNAL

LONDON SATURDAY JULY 3 1948

A MESSAGE TO THE MEDICAL PROFESSION

FROM THE MINISTER OF HEALTH

On July 5 we start, together, the new National Health Service. It has not had an altogether trouble-free gestation! There have been understandable anxieties, inevitable in so great and novel an undertaking. Nor will there be overnight any miraculous removal of our more serious shortages of nurses and others and of modern replanned buildings and equipment. But the sooner we start, the sooner we can try together to see to these things and to secure the improvements we all want.

On July 5 there is no reason why the whole of the doctor-patient relationship should not be freed from what most of us feel should be irrelevant to it, the money factor, the collection of fees or thinking how to pay fees—an aspect of practice already distasteful to many practitioners. Yet it has been vital, if this is to be the new situation, to see that it did not carry with it either any discouragement of professional and scientific freedom or any unfair worsening of a doctor's material livelihood. I sincerely hope and believe we have secured these things. If we have not we can easily put that right.

The picture I have always visualized is one, not of "panel doctoring" for the less well-off, not of anything charitable or demeaning, but rather of a nation deciding to make health-care easier and more effective by pooling its resources—each sharing the cost as he can through regular taxation and otherwise while he is well, and each able to use the resulting resources if and when he is ill. There is nothing of the social group or class in this; and I know you will be with me in seeing that there does not unintentionally grow up any kind of differentiation between those who use the new arrangements and those who, for any reason of their own, do not. Let this be a truly national effort. And I, for my part, can assure you that I shall want vigilantly to watch that your own intellectual and scientific freedom is never at risk of impairment by the background administrative framework, which has to be there for organizing purposes, but in which your own active participation is already secure.

In this comprehensive scheme—quite the most ambitious adventure in the care of national health that any country has seen—it will inevitably be you, and the other professions with you, on whom everything depends. My job is to give you all the facilities, resources, apparatus, and help I can, and then to leave you alone as professional men and women to use your skill and judgment without hindrance. Let us try to develop that partnership from now on.

It remains only to wish you all good luck, relief—as experience of the scheme grows—from your lingering anxieties, and a sense of real professional opportunity. I wish you them all, most cordially.

ANEURIN BEVAN

THANKS

With abundant thanks to all my colleagues who work within the NHS, clinical and non-clinical, many of whom worked through the Covid pandemic at great personal cost to themselves and their families.

For many months now I've greeted them with a question: if you were to magically become both Health Secretary and Chancellor of the Exchequer tomorrow, what would you do to fix the NHS? Their answers are woven throughout the text of this book, and though not all of them are acknowledged here, they know who they are and how grateful I am.

Particular thanks go to Julie Craig, Fiona Wright, Ishbel White, Christina Stitt, Claire Gall, Janis Blair, Jenna Pemberton, Pearl Ferguson, Sharon Lawson, Nicola Gray, Lynsay McDonald, Geraldine Fraser, John Dunn, Roy Robertson, Keith Taylor, Colin Speight, Bean Dhaun, Sam Guglani, Kate Womersley, Anna Dover and Robert Hunter. Thanks also to the energy and enthusiasm of my agent, Jenny Brown, and my publishers at Profile Books and the Wellcome Collection – Andrew Franklin, Penny Daniel, Cecily Gayford, Francesca Barrie, Valentina Zanca, Rosie Parnham, Susanne Hillen and Georgia Poplett.

Some passages within the text of this book have appeared in other publications, in other contexts, and I gratefully acknowledge the permission of their editors to include them here. I'm glad to have had the chance to bring them together in this new context, updated and extended, as part of a defence of the principles of the NHS.

To Paul Laity, who published my reflections on private medicine in the *Guardian Review* of 2 October 2015.

To Robbie Millen of *The Times* for permitting me to tell again the story of 'Agnes' in chapter 6, and for whom I reviewed James Le Fanu's *Too Many Pills* on 19 May 2018.

To Mary-Kay Wilmers, Jean McNicol and Alice Spawls, editors of the *London Review of Books*, who published my reflections on frailty, social care, over-diagnosis and overtreatment in the *LRB* of 5 March 2015 ('Cash for Diagnoses') and 2 March 2017 ('Diary').

To Tom Gatti of the *New Statesman* who published my review of Jeremy Hunt's memoir *Zero* on 30 May 2022.

And to Jonathan Beckman who published my reflections on the normalisation of crises in the NHS on 9 January 2023 in *1843 magazine* © The Economist Newspaper Limited, London, 2023. Parts of that piece have made their way into several sections of this book. Without the nudge from Jonathan I may not have embarked on writing *Free For All*. If the book makes even a modest difference to the way its readers think about the NHS, both its problems and some potential solutions, then it will have been worthwhile.

NOTES ON SOURCES

Online resources below all accessed June 2023.

1. A Day in the Life of (potentially) the Best Job in the World

p. 9, 'What is not so obvious ...', Aneurin Bevan, Chapter 5, *In Place of Fear* (London: William Heinemann, 1952)

p. 15, 'While hospital doctor numbers ...', Phil Whitaker, *What is a Doctor?* (Edinburgh: Canongate, 2023)

p. 15, 'the number of appointments offered ...', https://www.rcgp.org.uk/News/GP-appointments

p. 18, 'The current algorithms used ...', Whitaker, *What is a Doctor?*

2. In Place of Fear: The Origins of the NHS

p. 22, 'One of the steepest drops ...'. The UK figure for child mortality before the age of five today is 1 in 250; https://www.statista.com/statistics/1041714/united-kingdom-all-time-child-mortality-rate/

p. 22, 'By 2022 more people were dying ...', Danny Dorling, 'Fear', in *Shattered Nation* (London: Verso, 2023)

p. 23, 'By 1990 it had dropped ...', Dorling, 'Fear', in
    Shattered Nation

p. 25, 'Society becomes more wholesome ...', Aneurin
    Bevan, *In Place of Fear* (London: William Heinemann,
    1952)

p. 26, 'The service guaranteed ...',
    https://60yearsofnhsscotland.co.uk/history/birth-of-
    nhs-scotland/highlands-and-islands-medical-service.
    html

p. 26, 'The recruitment and retention of staff ...', https://
    www.uclan.ac.uk/news/new-research-exposes-scale-of-
    healthcare-inequalities-in-rural-communities-1

p. 29, 'Those first few years ...' Aneurin Bevan, *In Place of
    Fear*

p. 31, Some are undoubtedly too large 'to admit of good
    doctoring': https://www.ncbi.nlm.nih.gov/pmc/
    articles/PMC3750799/ from 2013, and https://www.ncbi.
    nlm.nih.gov/pmc/articles/PMC7643819/, 2020

p. 31, 'Amazingly enough, patients who ...', https://bjgp.
    org/content/72/715/e84

p. 33, What matters most ...', Alison Hill and George
    Freeman, 'Promoting Continuity of Care in General
    Practice', RCGP Policy Paper, March 2011

p. 33, 'There is a sound case ...', Bevan, *In Place of Fear*

p. 35, 'Those health services are as ...', https://www.
    health.org.uk/news-and-comment/news/uk-spent-
    around-a-fifth-less-than-european-neighbours-on-
    health-care-in-last-decade

p. 35, 'Just 2 per cent of the NHS workforce ...', https://

www.kingsfund.org.uk/publications/health-and-social-care-england-myths

p. 36, 'For too long the UK has relied …', https://www.commonwealthfund.org/publications/fund-reports/2021/aug/mirror-mirror-2021-reflecting-poorly#rank

p. 36, 'The NHS showed pockets …', https://www.bmj.com/content/367/bmj.l6326

3. The Normalisation of Crisis: No Slack in the System

p. 38, 'Public satisfaction with the NHS …', https://www.kingsfund.org.uk/publications/public-satisfaction-nhs-social-care-2021

p. 39, 'The NHS has stood …', Jeremy Hunt, *Zero: Eliminating Preventable Harm and Tragedy in the NHS* (London: Swift Press, 2022)

p. 40, 'if the people have willed …'; Powell quoted in Isabel Hardman, *Fighting for Life: The Twelve Battles that Made our NHS, and the Struggle for its Future* (London: Penguin Books, 2023), p. 61

p. 41, 'Illness is neither …', T. H. Marshall, *Social Policy in the Twentieth Century* (London: Hutchinson, 1965)

p. 42, 'They must bear in mind …', https://www.gmc-uk.org/news/news-archive/supporting-doctors-in-the-event-of-a-covid19-epidemic-in-the-uk

p. 42, 'The past few years …', https://www.gmc-uk.org/news/news-archive/winter-pressures---letter-to-the-profession

p. 45, 'we in the UK have fallen …', https://www.

kingsfund.org.uk/projects/health-and-social-care-bill/
mythbusters/nhs-performance

p. 45, 'The number of people who are ...', https://www.
kingsfund.org.uk/projects/public-satisfaction-nhs

p. 45, 'By 2022 there were 1.6 million ...' Dorling, *Shattered Nation*, pp. 163–64

p. 46, 'The NHS now needs upwards ...', https://www.
kingsfund.org.uk/blog/2016/01/how-does-nhs-
spending-compare-health-spending-internationally

p. 46, 'The then CEO of NHS England ...', https://www.
bbc.co.uk/news/health-56945830

p. 48, 'We already have among the lowest ...', https://
www.bma.org.uk/advice-and-support/nhs-delivery-
and-workforce/pressures/nhs-hospital-beds-data-
analysis

p. 48, 'Former NHS England chief Simon ...', https://
www.kingsfund.org.uk/publications/simon-stevens-
speaks-out-over-nhs-funding

p. 48, 'A year earlier Stevens had warned ...', https://bjgp.
org/content/68/672/308#ref-1

p. 49, 'In my area ...', https://www.nhslothian.scot/
yourrights/health-rights-waiting-times/nhs-lothian-
outpatient-waiting-times/

p. 50, 'I never want to ...', https://www.bbc.co.uk/news/
uk-scotland-65039689

p. 51, 'I am angry with every ...', Jonathan Lis interview
with Rachel Clarke, *Perspective Magazine*, 8 February
2023

p. 51, 'There is a huge amount of goodwill …', https://
www.bbc.com/news/uk-scotland-65039689

p. 52, 'Practices all around my own …'. For practices
closing their lists see https://www.edinburghnews.
scotsman.com/health/edinburgh-gp-crisis-six-practices-
close-to-new-patients-with-fears-issue-getting-worse-
with-no-end-in-sight-3949075; and for practices closing
altogether see this one from late 2022, Gracemount
Medical Practice, https://bidstats.uk/tenders/2022/
W45/786563414

p. 54, 'My profession of general practice …', https://
www.gmc-uk.org/about/what-we-do-and-why/data-
and-research/the-state-of-medical-education-and-
practice-in-the-uk/workforce-report-2022

p. 54, 'older and frailer than it has ever been …', https://
www.ons.gov.uk/peoplepopulationandcommunity/
populationandmigration/populationestimates/articles/
overviewoftheukpopulation/july2017

p. 54, 'As calls go out to …', https://www.mirror.co.uk/
news/uk-news/uks-least-accessible-gp-surgeries-
28572752

p. 54, 'they can only just cope with …', https://www.rcgp.
org.uk/News/GP-appointments

4. Workforce: We're All on the Same Team

p. 60, 'The availability of good medical care …'; see
https://www.thelancet.com/journals/lancet/article/
PIIS0140-6736(71)92410-X/fulltext

p. 60, 'Medical students who grew up ...', https://link.springer.com/article/10.1186/s12909-016-0536-1

p. 63, 'On the eve of the pandemic ...', https://www.rcn.org.uk/news-and-events/Press-Releases/vacancy

p. 64, 'In 2022 nurses were being paid ...', https://www.rcn.org.uk/news-and-events/news/uk-severe-nursing-workforce-shortages-new-rcn-report-exposes-urgent-need-for-government-action041122

p. 65, 'The suicide risk for healthcare workers ...', https://www.ons.gov.uk/peoplepopulationandcommunity/birthsdeathsandmarriages/deaths/articles/suicidebyoccupation/england2011to2015#main-points

p. 65, 'Doctors also have higher ...', https://bjgp.org/content/68/669/168.short

p. 65, 'which are also on the ...', https://www.bmj.com/content/349/bmj.g4839

p. 70, 'If the Service could be killed ...', Bevan, *In Place of Fear*

p. 70, 'Failing services are unhappy ...', https://www.theguardian.com/society/2022/mar/03/staffing-crisis-deepens-in-nhs-england-with-110000-posts-unfilled

p. 71, 'Can we really afford ...', https://www.bbc.com/news/uk-scotland-65039689

p. 77, 'When someone becomes ...', Whitaker, *What Is A Doctor?*

5. Patients or Shareholders? The Realities of Commercial Medicine

p. 80, 'The price of drugs ...', Karen Hassell, Vincenzo

Atella, Ellen I. Schafheutle, Marjorie C. Weiss, Peter R. Noyce, 'Cost to the patient or cost to the healthcare system? Which one matters the most for GP prescribing decisions?' *European Journal of Public Health*, 13(1), 2003, pp. 18–23

p. 85, 'Private hospitals are there …', Andrew Lees, *Brainspotting: Adventures in Neurology* (Kendal: Notting Hill Editions, 2022)

p. 87, 'many of the companies who won …', https://www.nhsforsale.info/gps/contract-failures-gps/

p. 90, 'Independent hospitals …', Hunt, *Zero*

p. 94, 'In another GMC survey …'. See MD, *Private Eye*, May 2023.

p. 95, 'Prepared he was …', *Canterbury Tales*, Prologue, lines 427–30

p. 95, 'avareis', *A Dictionary of the Older Scottish Tongue*, William A. Craigie (Chicago: University of Chicago Press, 1937)

p. 96, 'One must not be anxious …', Hippocrates, *Precepts* 4, Loeb Classical Library

6. Too Much Medicine: Overtreatment and Overdiagnosis

p. 105, 'up to 10 per cent of emergency …', James Le Fanu, *Too Many Pills* (London: Little, Brown, 2018)

p. 107, 'fatal heart attack by 27 per cent …', J. Shepherd , M. Cobbe, I. Ford et al., 'Prevention of coronary heart disease with pravastatin in men with hypercholesterolemia' (for the West of Scotland

Coronary Prevention Study Group), *The New England Journal of Medicine*, 333, 1995, pp. 1301–07

p. 108, 'tighter control conferred ...', Le Fanu, *Too Many Pills*

p. 109, 'We have found no ...', Lindsay Forbes, 'Review of the Quality and Outcomes Framework in England', Policy Research Unit in Commissioning and the Healthcare System, December 2016

p. 115, 'at the time of writing they cost ...', https://www.neurologylive.com/view/biogen-50-percent-drop-aducanumab-price-feedback-costs

p. 117, 'Regular infusions of a drug ...', https://www.england.nhs.uk/2019/05/nhs-england-strikes-deal-to-make-innovative-multiple-sclerosis-drug-available-paving-the-way-for-nice-recommendation/

p. 117, 'was at one point the most expensive ...', https://www.england.nhs.uk/2018/10/nhs-set-to-save-150-million-by-switching-to-new-versions-of-most-costly-drug/

p. 120, 'These "QALYS" ...', https://bmchealthservres.biomedcentral.com/articles/10.1186/s12913-020-5050-9

p. 121, 'The list price of £2.8 million ...', https://www.bbc.co.uk/news/health-60245738

p. 121, 'the body NHS Improvement ...', https://www.nhsconfed.org/publications/202223-nhs-priorities-and-operational-planning-guidance

p. 122, 'the taxpayer spends ...', https://www.kingsfund.org.uk/publications/rising-cost-medicines-nhs

p. 122, 'having access to a GP costs ...', https://www.bma.

org.uk/advice-and-support/nhs-delivery-and-
workforce/funding/investment-in-general-practice

7. Frailty and Social Care: A Magnificent Success Story

p. 124, 'Before the Covid dip …', https://ourworldindata.
org/life-expectancy

p. 125, 'in terms of costs to the NHS …', https://www.bbc.
co.uk/news/health-42572110

p. 125, 'It's between the ages of …', https://www.statista.
com/statistics/681523/individuals-with-private-health-
insurance-in-the-united-kingdom/

p. 127, 'One day extra in hospital …', https://www.ncbi.nlm.
nih.gov/pmc/articles/PMC7045184/

p. 137, https://qni.org.uk/news-and-events/news/district-
nurse-workforce-under-threat/

8. Identifying Problems, Exploring Solutions

p. 139, 'a bill to the taxpayer that …', https://www.bbc.
co.uk/news/business-42724939

p. 140, 'leaving a £9 billion backlog …', https://www.
kingsfund.org.uk/projects/nhs-in-a-nutshell/nhs-
capital-investment

p. 140, 'My job is to give you …', Aneurin Bevan, 'A
Message to the Medical Profession', *British Medical
Journal*, 3 July 1948

p. 141, 'defunding the service, neglectful …', Hunt, *Zero*

p. 151, 'If you're lucky, you can get away …', https://www.
ft.com/content/b2154c20-c9d0-4209-9a47-95d114d31f2b

p. 152, 'The budget for the NHS in England …', https://

www.england.nhs.uk/publications/business-plan/our-2022-23-business-plan/our-funding/

p. 152, 'For all claims, legal costs ...', https://www.gov.uk/government/news/new-cap-on-legal-costs-to-save-nhs-500-million

p. 154, 'New Zealand has an entirely ...', https://www.commonwealthfund.org/publications/journal-article/2006/feb/no-fault-compensation-new-zealand-harmonizing-injury

p. 156, 'He comes into...', Bevan, *In Place of Fear*

9. Save Our Service

p. 159, 'On 5 July we start ...', Bevan, 'A Message to the Medical Profession'

p. 165, 'within a few years ...', Chris Ham, *The Rise and Decline of the NHS in England 2000–20*, King's Fund report April 2023

wellcome collection

WELLCOME COLLECTION publishes thought-provoking books exploring health and human experience, in partnership with leading independent publisher Profile Books.

WELLCOME COLLECTION is a free museum and library that aims to challenge how we think and feel about health by connecting science, medicine, life and art, through exhibitions, collections, live programming, and more. It is part of Wellcome, a global charitable foundation that supports science to solve urgent health challenges, with a focus on mental health, infectious diseases and climate.

wellcomecollection.org